TESTIMONIALS

I was a skinny kid who started gaining weight in my early teens. I struggled to control it unsuccessfully for forty years before I found *The Metabolism Miracle*. I had tears in my eyes reading through the book initially because Diane was the first person to perfectly capture my personal experiences with food and weight. I felt better within the first week when my energy soared and my pants became looser. Four years later I am maintaining a *weight loss of over thirty pounds and four sizes,* despite all the physical challenges I experience with rheumatoid arthritis. Cravings and emotional eating are gone, and I embrace every new day with hope for a healthy future.

—*Nancy Rosati, New Jersey*

I was diagnosed with metabolic syndrome almost fifteen years ago. The only advice I was given was to "watch my diet." So I tried to eat healthy and watched as my cholesterol, blood glucose, blood pressure, and weight continued to rise. I ate less and exercised more. Watched as others ate what they wanted and maintained their weight. In January of 2013, after a desperate Internet search, I found *The Metabolism Miracle*. I thought, well, why not? I'll give this a try, and when it doesn't work I can legitimately say nothing works for me. That was *fifty pounds and four dress sizes ago.* My blood work is great and I feel wonderful!

—*Brenda Cash, Kansas*

I'd been overweight my entire life, and at one time or another, I tried most of the popular diets. If I lost anything on them, the pounds would soon yo-yo back, plus a few more. I have always exercised and also have a very physical job. Even with my exercise and physical work, I continued to gain fat.

D0210517

I started MM in June of 2012, exercising moderately for at least thirty minutes over and above my normal activity. In August I ramped up my exercise intensity. This increased exercise intensity helped me to reach a nontypical loss of inches based on the pounds I lost—*twenty-one pounds of fat and 39.5 inches!* Muscle is very condensed, tight, toned tissue, and losing close to 40 inches made an enormous difference in the way I look.

Since I've been blessed with no major health issues, my original MM goal was to lose weight. But what has transpired is so much more than pounds lost on a scale. The Metabolism Miracle has become a lifestyle that I can live for a lifetime and feel, look, and become healthy. I no longer have cravings or food binges, and I am in control of my food intake. Natural peanut butter and an evening cocktail allowed—real life!

—*Dee Grahl, Wisconsin*

The Metabolism Miracle is working around the world! I am in South Africa. Battling with high blood pressure (four blood pressure pills every day), I was also very overweight, unhealthy, and suffering from asthma. My pulmonologist asked me if he could suggest a book to me . . . it was *The Metabolism Miracle!* Since then my life changed. I lost over sixty-one pounds in the first year, I'm down to one blood pressure pill, my asthma is controlled, and I am full of energy! Previously I was too tired to walk in the shopping mall; now I am "running" through the mall. Thank you, Diane Kress! Your program saved my life.

—*Amanda Potgieter, South Africa*

The
Metabolism
Miracle

ALSO BY DIANE KRESS

The Metabolism Miracle Cookbook

The Diabetes Miracle

The
Metabolism
Miracle

3 Easy Steps to Regain Control
of Your Weight ... Permanently

Diane Kress, RD CDE

Da Capo
LIFE
LONG

A Member of the Perseus Books Group

Second Da Capo Press edition 2016

Published by Da Capo Press
A Member of the Perseus Books Group
www.dacapopress.com

Library of Congress Cataloging-in-Publication Data
Names: Kress, Diane, author.
Title: The metabolism miracle : 3 easy steps to regain control of your weight. permanently / by Diane Kress.
Description: Second edition. | Boston, MA : Da Capo Lifelong Books, a member of the Perseus Books Group, [2016] | Includes bibliographical references and index.
Identifiers: LCCN 2016006388 (print) | LCCN 2016011367 (ebook) | ISBN 9780738218908 (paperback) | ISBN 9780738218915 (ebook)
Subjects: LCSH: Weight loss. | Metabolism—Regulation. | BISAC: HEALTH & FITNESS / Diets. | HEALTH & FITNESS / Healthy Living.
Classification: LCC RM222.2 .K75 2016 (print) | LCC RM222.2 (ebook) | DDC 613.2/5—dc23
LC record available at http://lccn.loc.gov/2016006388

Note: The information in this book is true and complete to the best of our knowledge. This book is intended only as an informative guide for those wishing to know more about health issues. In no way is this book intended to replace, countermand, or conflict with the advice given to you by your own physician. The ultimate decision concerning care should be made between you and your doctor. We strongly recommend you follow his or her advice. Information in this book is general and is offered with no guarantees on the part of the authors or Da Capo Press. The authors and publisher disclaim all liability in connection with the use of this book.

Da Capo Press books are available at special discounts for bulk purchases in the U.S. by corporations, institutions, and other organizations. For more information, please contact the Special Markets Department at the Perseus Books Group, 2300 Chestnut Street, Suite 200, Philadelphia, PA, 19103, or call (800) 810-4145, ext. 5000, or e-mail special.markets@perseusbooks.com.

Editorial production by *Marrathon* Production Services. www.marrathon.net

Book design by Jane Raese
Set in 11-point Avance

LSC-C

10 9 8 7 6 5 4 3

This book is dedicated with love and gratitude to

my greatest inspirations

JC, Therese, Phil, Diana, Phillip, Jay, Jennifer, Jason, and Joey

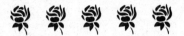

Contents

Diane Kress on
The Metabolism Miracle, Second Edition

As *The Metabolism Miracle, Second Edition* is published, I am in my thirty-fifth year as a registered dietitian (RD), medical nutritionist, and certified diabetes educator (CDE). Throughout my career I have specialized in medical nutrition therapy for those struggling with weight and obesity, PCOS, metabolic syndrome, prediabetes, and type 2 diabetes.

During the first fifteen years of my career I worked for and eventually directed nutrition programs at hospital-based diet centers, including medical nutrition therapy, weight loss, and diabetes. The American Dietetic Association (now the Academy of Nutrition and Dietetics) sanctioned the diet programs at these centers. While I worked within the association-approved diet parameters with my patients, I simultaneously collected data on any changes in their body weight, body measurements, blood pressure, nutrition-related lab data, and medications. I was expecting to track the fruits of their labor. Amazingly, however, my data continually showed that long-term success was practically nonexistent for the vast majority of patients.

Most of my RD and MD colleagues felt certain these unsuccessful patients weren't "doing as they were taught." I was convinced that almost all of our patients could not be failing in their effort to follow their diet program, and, instead, perhaps the diet protocol we unquestioningly taught might be failing our patients.

As if to confirm my suspicions, one day I had to count myself among the "patients" who carefully embraced and lived within the recommended diet protocol only to find myself gaining weight, acquiring medical conditions, and requiring medications.

After fifteen years of teaching "by the book," I could no longer ignore the disturbing data. Meticulous data collection proved that most patients regained any lost weight; eventually required medication, with increasing doses and types; and reported feeling depressed, anxious, and frustrated with their "no win" situation.

Looking closely at the trends in weight, body measurements, labs, medications, and symptoms, I realized there was a common denominator in patients who could not lose weight and get healthy on traditional diet methodology. It became painfully clear that many—most—of the patients counseled for weight loss, metabolic syndrome, PCOS, pre-diabetes, and diabetes could not succeed on the calorie-based and low-fat program the medical associations promoted.

I spent countless hours analyzing the standard diets, dissecting their components to expose the bare bones. I focused on how the "normal healthy body" processes, digests, absorbs, and metabolizes food. In the process I realized not all bodies process food the same way, not all bodies are "textbook." If certain people processed food differently and had metabolisms that worked differently from what was traditionally believed, it followed that the textbook low-calorie, low-fat diet would not work for everyone.

I could no longer instruct patients on diet programs I knew were destined to fail them. I decided to take a giant leap outside the box of medically recommended protocol. On that life-changing day I walked out the door of the hospital's diet center and into my own private practice.

Over the next several years I worked with thousands of patients, collected data, refined my new program, and was finally satisfied that I had developed a diet protocol that really did what it promised to do. The finished product enabled permanent weight loss and improved weight-related health conditions as well as energy and quality of life.

After years of refining and tweaking this state-of-the-science method of losing weight, keeping it off, and attaining and maintaining health and wellness, I wrote my first book, *The Metabolism Miracle*.

The Metabolism Miracle was specifically designed to match the metabolism of those with alternate metabolism—those who do not process and metabolize food according to the textbooks. As it turned out, about

60 percent of the US population has this "alternative" way of processing and metabolizing food.

The program has been successful from the beginning and will always be the recommended lifestyle—diet and exercise program—for the majority of adults who find they are unable to lose weight and keep it off. It is based in real science, human anatomy and physiology, and the way some peoples' metabolism progressively changes over a lifetime of stressors. The medical community is slowly but surely agreeing with the program's principles. Calories in–calories out, low-calorie, low-fat dieting is *not* for everyone. A person's genetic makeup plus a lifetime of environmental stressors can cause the majority of adults to overprocess the nutrient *carbohydrate*, making it impossible for them to lose weight, keep it off, and get and remain healthy on a regular diet.

This revised edition of *The Metabolism Miracle* offers new explanations, changes, tips, tricks, and tweaks that make the original program easier to follow and even more understandable, and it brings the program up-to-date regarding the latest research and new food products. You'll also find brand-new recipes, including easy, one-serving recipes for when you're cooking for yourself.

I am certain you will appreciate the latest fine-tuning of this excellent program. You *will* succeed in losing weight and fat, keeping it off, attaining and maintaining better health, and looking and feeling younger and more energetic for years to come.

Wishing you the very best,
Diane Kress

The Metabolism Miracle Commitment Contract

This is the Metabolism Miracle Commitment Contract. When you sign your name and commit to this contract, you are more likely to follow the program to the best of your ability.

If you ever feel like going off-program, reread the contract you signed *before* you make that decision. Reading aloud the words of your commitment contract may help you focus and find the strength to stay committed to MM.

The Metabolism Miracle Commitment Contract

Today I commit to the Metabolism Miracle lifestyle program.

- ✓ I understand and respect that I have Metabolism B and that *The Metabolism Miracle* is written for my specific metabolic needs.
- ✓ I will follow MM's steps in order, beginning with a minimum of eight weeks of Step One.
- ✓ I will weigh myself and get all body measurements at the start and end of every eight-week period (with time added for slip-ups).
- ✓ I will find my "expected weight/inch loss" in the book, and at the end of eight weeks (plus time added for slip-ups) I will compare lost pounds and inches to my starting weight and inches. If I'm not in my target range for pounds and inches lost or if pounds and inches lost are not within two points of each other, I will recheck the instructions in the book or through a food-log analysis, available on the subscription support site at www.Miracle-Ville.com.
- ✓ I know that the recommended physical activity, fluids, vitamins/supplements, green tea (optional), adequate rest, and stress management are necessary for a healthy life and vow to follow the entire program for best results.

_____

(name)   *(today's date)*

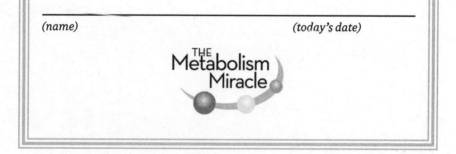

Introduction

The Metabolism Miracle:
A Simple yet Effective Lifestyle Program
Developed for *Your* Metabolic Needs

In over thirty-five years, having worked directly with tens of thousands of patients, clients, and readers, I've met many frustrated dieters. They sit across the desk from me at my private practice, meet me after a lecture, and speak with me through the MM support site, Miracle-Ville .com. They most often tell me that the Metabolism Miracle will be their last attempt to lose weight: "If this program doesn't work, I am giving up."

Diet after diet, pounds lost, pounds regained—they are tired of trying. They've given up many times before, tried so many programs, and faced so many broken promises. Despite their investment in focus, time, money, energy, and work, they never attain lasting results.

That all changes with the Metabolism Miracle.

Diets are built on the assumption that everyone's metabolism works in the same way and that a diet that works for one person will work equally for another. In other words, metabolism is metabolism, and one size fits all. But what if your metabolism doesn't quite match the textbook version? What if your body works a little differently from what was presumed? What if you weren't failing at dieting, but instead your diet was failing you?

In fact, over 60 percent of people I've worked with for weight loss and weight-related health issues as well as millions of people across the country and worldwide really do have a very different metabolism from what was thought to be "standard metabolism." These frustrated people can start diet after diet and faithfully follow the rules that produced results for their friends. Unbeknownst to them, all previous weight-loss programs and books could no longer work for them because these books were written to match what was considered to be the "standard metabolism," but their metabolism had progressed to Metabolism B.

If you find it impossible to lose weight and keep it off, even when you follow all the rules, there's an excellent chance your metabolism no longer matches the cookie-cutter metabolism. The Metabolism Miracle is designed for people like you and will help you understand your body and learn to live with it rather than against it.

The Metabolism Miracle is not just another diet book. The program is the result of thirty-five years of working with thousands of patients whose metabolism did not follow the expected norm. Before I discovered the way to fuel this metabolism properly, those whose metabolism had morphed into Metabolism B had little to no chance of permanent weight loss, no matter how hard they tried. Now they have the potential for 100 percent success.

Be Prepared to Be Surprised

On any given day, between 25 and 35 percent of Americans over the age of twenty are actively trying to lose weight. When polled, over 60 percent of US adults report knowing they are either overweight or obese. (According to the National Institutes of Health [NIH], 69 percent of the adult population is overweight or obese.[1])

Despite all the news, press, advertised weight-loss programs, weight-loss products and aids, and backing by the machinery of a multibillion-dollar weight-loss industry, a 2013 Gallup poll found that Americans' eating habits are, in fact, worsening.[2]

For those who are actively trying to lose or maintain weight loss following popular diets, recommended diets, fad diets, or even physician-ordered diets, I can only imagine the frustration you feel as you lose a few pounds, regain them, lose a little again, and then regain it all. The roller-coaster ride of up-and-down weight is enough to frustrate anyone.

The world is becoming sicker as a consequence. Many serious health conditions are linked directly to being overweight or obese. The risk of developing type 2 diabetes, cardiovascular disease, cancer, hypertension, acid reflux disease, sleep apnea, and depression increases as weight gain progresses.

In fact, 65 percent of dieters who have managed to lose weight will regain all of it within three years, while 95 percent will regain all of the weight they lost within five years. That means the long-term success rate of any of the available diets is a meager 5 percent—only five out of one hundred serious dieters have been able to maintain their weight loss.[3] As a result, people become desperate, jumping from diet to diet, even undergoing weight-loss surgery, hoping to find the magic formula that will help them lose unhealthy weight and keep it off for a lifetime. And when they are not successful, they feel *they* did not do a good job and have failed in losing weight and keeping it off.

Even the high-profile diet programs pay celebrities to be spokespersons during their advertising campaigns, especially during the "New Year New You" campaign, hiring the same "celebrities" over and over. A celebrity spokesperson will promote the program, lose a great deal of weight very quickly, then regain every pound and come back to promote the program a few years later. Kirstie Alley, Oprah Winfrey, Dan Marino, Marie Osmond, Charles Barkley, and Chris Berman are only a handful of celebrity diet spokespeople who continue to lose weight, gain weight, lose weight, gain weight. They can afford to follow *any* weight-loss program, have a chef to prepare all their meals and snacks, have someone shop for their food supplies, have a trainer for exercise—and still they fail on the diet they gushed about.

The Metabolism Miracle breaks through this dieting madness. For years medical science recognized a one-size-fits-all metabolism and promoted diet and weight-loss programs based on how the medical community assumed all bodies handled food. More recently researchers identified an alternative metabolism and categorized it under a variety of terms, including metabolic syndrome, Syndrome *X*, insulin imbalance, and insulin resistance. Millions of people have this alternative metabolism, which I refer to as *Metabolism B*.

Unfortunately a lifetime lifestyle program has never been fully developed to work in tandem with all the special requirements of this different type of metabolism. Up until now there was no diet to rely upon for permanent weight loss.

If you have Metabolism B, you were born with a different blueprint for processing food. As your life progressed, your genetic makeup made it possible for *you* to acquire Met B.

As life presented more stressors, you may have noticed your inability to lose weight and keep it off. Tried-and-true diets no longer worked. You seemed to gain weight whether you ate, overate, or didn't eat.

Met B is a progressive condition, and everyone's tolerance to life stressors is different. At the time you began having difficulty losing excess weight, your Met B may have advanced to the point that you noticed some of its universal symptoms, including progressive weight gain around the middle (belly fat), fatigue, and carb cravings. Unchecked, the symptoms lead to health issues involving cholesterol, blood glucose, vitamin D, and blood pressure. Your body could no longer behave using the same diet rules that work for others. Instead, you now require a program that has been designed with your blueprint in mind.

The Metabolism Miracle program is a three-step approach that rests your body's overactive response to carbohydrate, then retrains your body to handle carbohydrate normally, and lastly enables you to live a life in harmony with your type of metabolism. Once you learn to live in balance with your metabolism, your excess weight will gradually come off and *permanently* stay off. Your health will improve, your energy level will soar, and you'll experience a feeling of peace and contentment. Miraculously, you will begin to feel the effects of this new approach in less than one week.

To determine whether you have Metabolism B, you will complete a basic checklist that pinpoints the telltale signs, symptoms, and personal medical history that characterize people with Metabolism B. If you would like more in-depth proof, your most recent fasting lab data can verify the results. Either way, your search for the right weight-loss program has ended.

The Metabolism Miracle will help you understand the way your body works and empower you to work with your metabolism instead of against it.

The Metabolism Miracle will bring back the healthy you—no more carb cravings, energy slumps, food binges, or frustrating weight regain. You will learn about the foods you can eat whenever you are hungry, with no calorie counting, weighing, or measuring. You'll also learn about the energy foods that will fuel your metabolism all day long. Weight-related health problems will diminish and even disappear. And you will feel healthier and more energized than you have felt in years or perhaps in your lifetime.

The Metabolism Miracle is easy, effective, and, best of all, the first and only program written expressly for *you*.

PART ONE

Your Metabolism Is Different

1

A Proven Program to Change Your Life

You know who you are.

You have suffered through liquid diets, portion-controlled diets, calorie counting, point counting, fat-free diets, carb-free diets, grapefruit diets, cabbage soup diets, and even medically supervised diets—only to regain every pound you lost. You sit at weight-loss support meetings next to people who succeed while you do not. You are truly an expert in dieting. You can recite the calorie content of foods without glancing at a book. You have tried, over and over. *You really have tried.*

Yet you have known for a long time that something is very different about your body. Others eat twice the quantity of food that you consume and weigh much less than you. No matter what the doctors and nutritionists say, you insist that you must have a different metabolism.

You are right.

I know this because, like you, I have this different metabolism, and it confounded me for many years of my life. The Metabolism Miracle is the culmination of my life's work in treating people with stubborn weight and weight-related issues.

The story of the Metabolism Miracle began with me. Even before I became a registered dietitian I knew there was something different about my body. Despite my best attempts at weight loss, I always regained every pound I lost, my energy was sapped, I felt older than my age, and I had difficulty with focus and concentration.

It took many years as a registered dietitian specializing in weight loss to find and acknowledge the problem. To date, I have spent more than thirty-five years as a registered dietitian specializing in weight loss, obesity, PCOS, metabolic syndrome, insulin imbalance, and type 2 diabetes.

But it wasn't until I put it all together based on my own and thousands of patients' weight-loss issues that I could clearly see the flaw in the standard diet. And this previously unrecognized diet flaw continues to impact approximately 60 percent of people trying to lose weight, keep it off, and get healthy.

The Metabolism Miracle changed my life and continues to change the lives and health of the millions of people who can't lose weight or keep it off without this program.

A Personal Story

As a registered dietitian, trained in the traditional approach to nutrition, I have counseled thousands of people over the years and worked equally hard with all of them. Yet early in my clinical practice I noticed something that deeply concerned me: more than 60 percent of those I counseled never achieved their desired results.

In the traditional school of thought a person will gain weight if he or she consumes more calories than are burned off. Most weight-loss diets are based on this "law of calories." The fewer calories a person consumes, the less he or she will weigh. Add physical activity to the equation, and weight loss accelerates. But what if the law of calories didn't apply to all people?

For years I used a universal formula, the Harris-Benedict equation, for all of my weight-loss clients to determine the number of calories they should consume in order to lose weight. I dutifully plugged my patients' gender, height, desired weight, age, and physical activity into the formula and came up with a calorie allotment that should have guaranteed their weight loss. If the patient's cholesterol was elevated, I added a saturated fat and dietary cholesterol restriction. If they suffered from hypertension, I added a sodium restriction. The formula then configured a nice, neat diet package with precise calorie allotments. This is the same diet many physicians, dietitians, and nutritionists provide today.

The patients followed the diet, weighed and measured food portions, kept detailed food journals, and exercised regularly. But many of them returned for their follow-up visit disillusioned and depressed: nothing significant had happened! They had lost little weight and had no real change in their blood lipids, blood sugar, or blood pressure. They remained on medications, and worse yet, their medications increased over the years.

I sympathized, but I also wondered whether they had truly followed my instructions. Perhaps they wrote what they believed I wanted to see in their food logs. Maybe, in reality, they didn't follow the plan or exercise. Perhaps they were overeating or sneaking in snacks. The diet worked for some of my clients, so why didn't it work for all of them?

As time passed I realized that if I were to help these patients, I would have to challenge some of the principles that the medical community had written in stone. There had to be a reason for the obesity epidemic. Why was type 2 diabetes afflicting more and younger people? Why were so few people succeeding at diets despite the billion-dollar weight-loss industry? Why were we becoming a nation reliant on prescription medications? Something had to be very wrong with the theories.

Then something alarming happened to me.

As a nutrition counselor with a thriving practice, I knew everything there was to know about diets; I could configure them in my sleep. I prided myself in following a balanced, healthful diet. I exercised regularly and practiced what I preached. But as I entered my thirties my body changed.

At a routine physical exam a nurse told me that my consistently low blood pressure had increased to the normal zone. Shortly after, my cholesterol and triglyceride levels began to rise, regardless of exercise and my low-calorie, low-fat, low-cholesterol lifestyle. Soon, even as I counted every calorie that passed my lips, the numbers on the scale began to creep upward. Worse yet, I noticed a roll of fat forming around my middle!

I followed the guidelines I had been taught were the key to good health. I lived the traditional, standard diet programs. Like my patients, I monitored my calories, fat, cholesterol, and sodium, and I exercised faithfully. Despite all of this effort, I continued to gain weight and eventually needed medication to help control my blood pressure and cholesterol.

Finally, just before my fortieth birthday, I developed type 2 diabetes. What had happened? It seemed as if nothing I did would stop this train!

Despite my attempts to do everything by the book, my body did not respond appropriately. I finally felt the full force of the frustration and emotional pain my patients endured.

The experience led me right back to the traditional nutrition theories I had been teaching my patients. I started to keep detailed data on their blood pressure, cholesterol, and blood glucose as they followed their diet program. I dug into the latest research on metabolism and weight loss. What was different about the patients who succeeded on the traditional diet and those who were unsuccessful? I tested different approaches, threw out those that didn't work, and came up with confirmation of what I had come to suspect: one segment of dieters responded to the traditional approach, but the others needed a very different and new approach. The Metabolism Miracle is that new approach.

The new program worked. Within the first few weeks on the program I felt like a new person, with higher energy, looser jeans, and no cravings. Within the second month my doctor eliminated my hypertension medication and decreased my medication for cholesterol. Eventually I no longer needed any of my medications, and my blood pressure, cholesterol, weight, and diabetes remained under good control! I felt great, and friends told me I looked ten years younger.

Not only did the program work for me; it worked for the patients who fit the profile for and followed this very different way of eating. There are definitely two very different styles of metabolism. In order to succeed losing weight and getting healthy for the long term, everyone needs to know their metabolic type to point them in the direction of the right diet and lifestyle plan for their body.

A Different Kind of Metabolism

Most weight-loss advice recognizes only one metabolism, the version every medical and dietetics student is familiar with. I refer to this "universally" recognized metabolism type as *Metabolism A*.

Weight-loss diets have traditionally been designed to work for those with Metabolism A, as the medical community assumed that we all have the same type of metabolism. Diets based on "calories in minus calories out," low in fat grams, with a focus on complex carbohydrates are designed for so-called normal metabolism, or Metabolism A (Met A).

If a person metabolizes food differently from the universally accepted Met A way, standard, traditional diets will not match their metabolism. Trying to follow a traditional weight-loss diet based on Metabolism A when a person has a different metabolism type is like trying to fit a square peg into a round hole—it simply won't work.

I failed to lose weight and retain my good health following standard diets designed for Metabolism A, and I watched so many of my patients go down the same path. I began to refer to our alternate metabolism as *Metabolism B (Met B)*. This alternative metabolism requires an entirely different approach for long-term weight loss and health benefits, and that is how the Metabolism Miracle began to take shape.

Before we discuss how to know if you have Metabolism A or Metabolism B, it is important to understand the term *metabolic syndrome*. Those who eventually develop metabolic syndrome have the genetic predisposition to Metabolism B.

Doctors first began to recognize metabolic syndrome way back in the 1920s. Not a single disease, metabolic syndrome is a cluster of health conditions. Think of Metabolism B as the precursor to metabolic syndrome. You are born with the genes for metabolic syndrome (Met B), but life's stressors cause it to manifest.

The National Institutes of Health has defined metabolic syndrome as a metabolic disorder in which a person has three or more of the following:

- a waist measuring at least forty inches for men and thirty-five inches for women
- triglycerides over 150 mg/dL
- HDL cholesterol less than 40 mg in men and less than 50 mg in women
- blood pressure of at least 135/80
- fasting blood glucose over 110 mg/dL

Simply put, the diagnosis of metabolic syndrome is based on such factors as being overweight, having a large waist circumference, high LDL (bad) cholesterol and triglycerides, low HDL (good) cholesterol, hypertension, and higher than normal blood glucose. When metabolic syndrome is diagnosed, the combination of genes and assorted lifestyle factors that include weight gain, inactivity, hormonal changes, high carbohydrate diet, certain medications, emotional stress, illness, and chronic pain are already present.

Dr. Margo Dente, professor of medicine at the University of Texas, noted that being able to identify metabolic syndrome can go a long way to improving it. "This is one syndrome that is exquisitely lifestyle-sensitive—it's an area where we can get people to pay attention and if they do pay attention, there are big rewards," she said.[1] And Drs. Melissa Conrad Stöppler and William C. Shiel point out the surprising prevalence of the syndrome. "Metabolic syndrome is quite common," they write. Approximately 32 percent of the total adult population of the United States has metabolic syndrome, and a full 40 percent of American adults over sixty are affected, while 85 percent of those with type 2 diabetes have metabolic syndrome.[2]

Although a patient may clearly have the lab work, weight distribution, and blood pressure to diagnose metabolic syndrome, most physicians and healthcare professionals fail to diagnose their patients. And although metabolic syndrome has been recognized for years, no diet prior to the Metabolism Miracle has ever covered *all* the contributing factors that force the progression of metabolic syndrome. The Metabolism Miracle takes the whole package of symptoms, labs, and weight issues into account, stops the fat-gain train in its tracks, and even helps to reverse some of the health consequences of this previously uncontrolled metabolic progression.

Individuals with Metabolism B will never succeed at following a traditional weight-loss diet based on lowering calories and increasing activity because their unique carbohydrate metabolism follows a different set of rules from those of the standard metabolism. In fact, attempting to lose weight using a traditional approach can set off the downward spiral of unchecked Metabolism B.

The split between dieters with Metabolism A and Metabolism B is slanted toward Met B. Over 60 percent of those struggling to lose weight are born with the genetic predisposition to Metabolism B. The onset of their symptoms is slow and progressive and may be expedited by a number of life events, including stress, weight gain, illness, and hormonal changes.

Take heart. You do not lack willpower! You are not a lazy dieter! You are not lying about what you eat or if you exercise! Your body simply responds to carbs differently from how science originally claimed. Once you understand your body, you can work with your unique metabolism instead of against it. By identifying whether you have Met A or Met B, you can easily make the right food choices to lead a healthy life at your healthy weight.

Because other diets haven't worked for people with Metabolism B, permanent weight loss can feel overwhelmingly difficult and often downright impossible. Add a health issue such as type 2 diabetes to the scenario, and the extra weight becomes downright scary. I know because I've been there.

If you have the genes that have set you up for a lifetime of struggles with weight, the Metabolism Miracle will absolutely work for you. Before the Metabolism Miracle, you had little to no chance of permanent weight loss. With this lifetime lifestyle program you can reach and maintain a healthy weight, your lab data will improve, the dose of medications you take to control weight-related health problems will decrease or disappear, and you may avoid health risks down the line.

Best of all, you will look and feel great!

2

Is This You?

Anyone can lose weight with the Metabolism Miracle, but the program is designed specifically for people who have Metabolism B—those who have a slim chance of long-term weight-loss success with any other diet plan. They will, for the first time, lose weight and *successfully* keep it off for the rest of their lives because this comprehensive lifestyle approach, unlike other weight-loss programs, matches their unique metabolism.

You may be thinking, *I must not have Metabolism B because only two years ago I could control my weight with no problem.* Keep in mind that people with Metabolism B have always had the genetic predisposition for this alternative metabolism, but it is only when outside triggers—such as emotional stress, weight gain, inactivity, hormonal changes, or illness—flip the switch that Metabolism B begins to manifest itself in symptoms such as weight gain around the middle, hypertension, or high cholesterol. Some people show symptoms as children, and others show symptoms during the teen or adult years. The longer a person has unknowingly lived with unchecked Metabolism B, the more progressive their weight gain and weight-related health issues become. (See Trouble Triggers, page 32.)

Thankfully, finding out whether you have Metabolism A or Metabolism B is very clear-cut.

To start, answer the following descriptive questions. Most people with Metabolism B see themselves as they answer *yes* to questions on the list. If you recognize yourself in a number of them, you may have Metabolism B and should move on to the easy personal symptoms checklists that follow. You can see the genetic link by looking at your family's medical history. Finally, if you've recently had fasting lab work done, you can see whether your lab work is consistent with uncontrolled Met B.

A Look in the Mirror

_____ Have you dieted for years, perhaps successfully in the past, but now even tried-and-true diets you once relied on for weight loss fail you?

_____ Do you notice that you can only stick to a diet for a short time and then the dismal results, constant hunger, and overwhelming cravings discourage you so much that you abandon your good intentions?

_____ Are you gaining weight regardless of your efforts, and is this weight shifting into a roll around your middle?

_____ Does the fat around your midsection look and feel spongy, loose, and watery?

_____ Can people around you eat more and yet weigh less than you?

_____ Is your overall health—physical, mental, and emotional—declining as your weight increases?

_____ Do you need medical prescriptions for weight-related health problems such as hypertension, cholesterol, triglycerides, acid reflux, insomnia, depression, anxiety, or arthritis pain?

_____ Despite diet and exercise, has your doctor been forced to increase your medication dosages or add new prescriptions to maintain your health?

_____ Do cravings sometimes gnaw at you like an addiction, and do you feel a strong urge to eat carbohydrates such as candy, sweets, bread, ice cream, pasta, or chips?

_____ Do you feel depressed, irritable, unattractive, and undesirable?

_____ Are you fatigued, even after a proper amount of sleep?

_____ Do you miss the "old you"?

_____ Do you look and feel older than you feel you should?

If you found yourself answering _yes_ to several of these questions, go directly to the following simple checklist of symptoms to learn whether the Metabolism Miracle can help you regain your health and well-being and enable permanent weight loss. If you answered _no_ to almost all of these checkpoints, it's quite possible that you have textbook metabolism, Metabolism A, and can lose weight on any good weight-loss program.

Clues to Metabolism B

This list of symptoms is one of the first pieces of information I use when trying to identify Metabolism A or Metabolism B. It still surprises me that when people with Metabolism A read the checklist, they only identify with a few of the symptoms, whereas people with Metabolism B relate to many if not most of them.

Check off any of the experiences that describe how you usually feel:

____ You are frequently fatigued, even upon awakening.

____ You feel mildly depressed.

____ You feel an energy slump in the late afternoon.

____ You frequently feel anxious and jumpy.

____ You crave carbohydrate foods—bread, chips, sweets, ice cream, pasta, fries, chocolate.

____ Your midsection has a roll of fat and the waist on your jeans is getting tighter.

____ You gain weight easily and find it difficult to lose weight.

____ You have trouble sleeping—falling asleep or staying asleep

____ You are often forgetful and worry about your short-term memory.

____ You have racing thoughts, even when you are in bed trying to fall asleep.

____ Your sex drive has declined. Along with a decreased libido, you may be experiencing erectile dysfunction (ED), frequent yeast infections, vaginal dryness, or feel too exhausted or disinterested to initiate sex.

____ You find it difficult to focus and concentrate and are easily distracted.

____ Bright light or headlights at night bother you.

____ You are irritable and have a "short fuse."

____ You have increased sensitivity to aches and pains.

____ Your eyes frequently tear up and at other times feel dry and irritated.

____ You get dull headaches, usually across your forehead.

_____ You feel slightly dizzy, flushed, or "weak in the knees" after even a small amount of alcohol.

_____ Coffee or caffeinated beverages have less of an impact.

If you have identified with many of the items on this symptoms checklist, you likely have Metabolism B.

You may have looked at the symptoms checklist for Metabolism B and thought they could be attributed to many different conditions, including menopause, chronic fatigue syndrome, getting older, dealing with a young family, or working a high-stress job. But at the end of eight weeks on Step One of the Metabolism Miracle many symptoms from the checklist will disappear along with weight because your symptoms stem from untreated Metabolism B.

If after eight weeks of Step One (plus time added for slip-ups), your symptoms persist, they are related to something else and should be addressed from another angle. For example, if after eight weeks a patient still has weight gain with no change in belly fat, it would be prudent to discuss this with his or her physician.

Blame It on the Genes

Certain medical conditions are very common in people with Metabolism B. They range from high cholesterol to type 2 diabetes. The longer you live without treating Metabolism B properly, the greater the chance you will develop an increasing number of these medical problems. The sooner you start the Metabolism Miracle, the more likely you are to avoid these problems in the future or, as is often the case, the more likely you can reverse them.

Many of these conditions work in a domino-like chain effect, with the genetic profile for Metabolism B starting the reaction. For example, it is Metabolism B's excessive insulin release that causes midline fat to accumulate. That midline fat in turn provokes insulin resistance, hypertension, and acid reflux (GERD). In another chain, excess insulin in the bloodstream promotes excess circulating fat such as cholesterol and triglycerides, and high levels of lipids in the blood in turn contribute to

"I'M JUST . . . OLD"

When I first met fifty-five-year-old Dee, she checked off almost all of the symptoms on the checklist. She handed the paper across the desk and said, "Of course I feel this way, Diane. I'm menopausal, have no time to exercise as I'm occupied with my work, a physical job that occupies long hours and leaves me spent. And, let's face it, I'm just . . . old."

I agreed the symptoms could relate to many conditions, but once people live the Metabolism Miracle lifestyle, they quickly discover that their uncontrolled Metabolism B may be to blame for many of the unpleasant symptoms.

Dee agreed to begin the three-step Metabolism Miracle lifestyle program but added that she didn't really believe it would work for her.

"I've tried every diet known to man, and nothing seems to budge this weight. Within a short time after I lose some weight I begin to regain pounds and end up heavier than when I started. With each diet failure I find myself looking older, feeling older, and getting very frustrated."

I next saw Dee at her nine-week follow-up visit. She was wearing fitted clothing and walked in with confidence. Her skin was glowing, her eyes were bright, and her shiny hair and overall demeanor made her look younger than her age.

"I've completed my first eight-week block of MM, and I'm a believer. Almost all those symptoms I had chalked up to age and my physically demanding job are totally gone or much improved. I have fewer mood swings, sleep soundly, have energy, and no cravings. I am much less forgetful and love that the waistline on my pants is getting looser."

When she stepped on the scale and I remeasured her, she had lost within her expected weight/inch range for this nine-week period and was ready to move to Step Two.

As she left the office she turned back. "It's funny, but one symptom hasn't improved yet. Actually, I still have aches and pains." After a short pause she continued, "Do you think these aches are from adding exercise to my already physically active days? For the first time in years I have the energy and motivation to exercise over and above my job activity, and my Zumba™ class uses very different muscles!"

coronary vascular disease. Fluctuating blood sugar levels, a direct result of unchecked Metabolism B, can contribute to mild depression, anxiety, panic attacks, and short-term memory loss. In time they can progress to prediabetes and type 2 diabetes. Hormonal imbalance can cause polycystic ovarian syndrome (PCOS), irregularity in menstrual cycles, and may even contribute to infertility. You get the picture.

If you are young and haven't experienced any of these conditions, don't wave them off. Remember, Metabolism B is a genetic syndrome. Look at your family's medical history, including your parents, siblings, grandparents, aunts, uncles, cousins. Have those family members manifested these health conditions?

Almost all of the medical conditions listed below will eventually require medication. When you fuel your metabolism correctly with a measured carbohydrate dose in the strategically timed pattern that is built into the Metabolism Miracle, the need for that medication may decline. You'll need less medication as you enjoy improved mental, physical, and emotional health as well as increased energy and weight loss.

If you've experienced any of the following medical conditions, you may want to read more about them and how they relate to your Metabolism B. For a detailed explanation of the following medical conditions, see the glossary.

Twenty-Six Health Conditions or Diseases That Are Directly Related to Insulin Imbalance and Uncontrolled Metabolism B
   atherosclerosis
   cancer (breast, colon, skin, uterus, ovaries, prostate)
   cardiovascular disease
   dementia/Alzheimer's disease
   depression and/or anxiety disorder and panic attacks
   elevated cholesterol
   elevated triglycerides
   GERD
   gestational diabetes
   heart attack
   high fasting insulin (8 or over)
   hypertension

hypoglycemia

inflammatory disease or auto-immune disease

insulin resistance

low vitamin D levels

metabolic syndrome

NAFLD (non-alcohol related fatty liver disease)

overweight/obesity

pancreatitis (non-alcohol related)

PCOS

prediabetes

sleep apnea or sleep disorders

stroke

type 2 diabetes

visceral fat (abdominal fat that builds around the stomach and
between organs)

If you identified with many of the clues on the symptoms checklist on page 12, you likely have Metabolism B. If, in addition, you or a close relative currently has or has had several of the above twenty-six medical conditions linked to Metabolism B, the case is even stronger for Metabolism B. Still skeptical? You may want to look at your most recent blood profile.

A Look at *Your* Numbers

It is not necessary to have lab work done before beginning the Metabolism Miracle program. But if you have had fasting blood work drawn within the past six months, compare your numbers to the Metabolism Miracle target ranges below. Keep in mind that the ranges used for this program are different from the American Medical Association and American Diabetes Association's current normal ranges because not only does MM help you keep off excess weight, it also focuses on preventing future medical problems. The lab work target ranges for Metabolism B will pinpoint your genetic disposition to Met B and enable you to make lifestyle changes to prevent its progression. Fasting lab work is required.

	Metabolism A	Metabolism B
Fasting blood glucose	65 to 85 inclusive	less than 65 mg/dL or greater than 85 mg/dL (less than 3.6 mmol/L or greater than 4.7 mmol/L
Fasting total cholesterol	less than 200	greater than 199 (greater than 5.2 mmol/L)
Fasting LDL cholesterol	less than 100	greater than 99 (greater than 2.6 mmol/L)
Fasting HDL cholesterol	greater than 45	less than 45 (less than 1.2 mmol/L)
Fasting cholesterol/HDL ratio	less than 5	5 or above
Fasting triglycerides	less than 100	less than 50 or greater than 99 (less than .6 mmol/L or greater than 1.1 mmol/L)
Fasting hemoglobin A1C	5.6 or less	less than 5.2 or greater than 5.6
Fasting blood pressure	less than 135/80	greater than 135/80
Fasting vitamin D	40 or over	less than 40
Fasting TSH	Between .45 and 4.5	less than .45 or greater than 4.5 mIU/L
Fasting insulin	Less than 8	Over 7.9

If you take medication to help control blood pressure, cholesterol, or blood sugar, your findings may *appear* in the normal range because they are being covered with a Band-Aid™ of medications. Ask yourself: *If I were not on medication, would these readings be normal?* Remember that this lab work needs to be drawn as *fasting* blood work (taken after at least eight hours without food or calorie-containing beverages).

Testing Fasting Insulin Level

Some program followers want proof that the program brings their insulin back into the normal range. If you don't wish to have a fasting insulin

I started MM at the end of June and had my initial blood tests done ten days later. Here are my starting numbers and my numbers four months later.

	July	November
A1C	12.8	6.5
Blood sugar	201	120
Lipids		
Total Cholesterol	182	161
Triglycerides	266	147
HDL	39	42
LDL	117	94

The nurse was absolutely amazed when she called me today, and I am tickled pink. I am still waiting to hear from the NP about what they will do with my meds.

I owe this to you, MM, and the support of Miracle-Ville!

—Beverly

test drawn, you can still determine that the pancreas and liver are rested at the end of every eight-week period if your weight/inches lost are in the expected fat/inch-loss range beginning on page 342.

For the objectivity of a blood test, ask your physician to consider ordering a fasting insulin level.

- Your fasting insulin level *after* eight or more weeks of Step One should be 6 or less
- Your fasting insulin level *after* eight weeks of Steps Two or Three should be 8 or less.

If you checked off a fasting glucose of 85 mg/dL or above, you most likely have Metabolism B and can rest assured that the Metabolism Miracle will work for you. The more lab results that are in the Met B range, the more influence Metabolism B has had on your health to this point. One of MM's goals is to get your lab work as close to normal as possible with as little medication as possible. In as little as eight weeks your physician may need to lower your dosage of medication as your body enters a healthier zone.

I thought I'd share my latest labs to hopefully encourage anyone just starting out or struggling. The weight loss is great—*sixty-eight pounds gone so far*—but my cardiologist originally suggested the Metabolism Miracle because my triglycerides were 637! My total cholesterol was over 300 and HbA1C was 8.9. Now, in just under a year, my triglycerides are 198, cholesterol 239, HbA1C is 5.6—approaching normal! I've stopped 90 percent of my meds with doctor recommendation. By next year this next sixty pounds should be gone along with the rest of my prescriptions. It really works!

—Becky S.

Finding the Hidden Health Clues

The first step when trying to decide which weight-loss/health-gain diet is right for you is to determine whether you have Met A or Met B. Without this clarification over 60 percent of all dieters will not be able to lose weight permanently because most weight-loss programs do not match their alternative metabolism.

Although each symptom, lab value, and personal and family medical history eventually adds up to a diagnosis of Met B, it is the sum total of check marks that equal the extent of the patient's metabolic story.

Belly Wars

Jason is a forty-two-year-old self-assured male who found himself in a serious battle with belly fat. Admittedly vain, Jason had been a star athlete in high school and college, still has a full head of wavy dark hair, and is considered a hunk in the workplace and neighborhood. He works hard as a financial adviser and is meticulous with his appearance.

Jason goes to the gym six days a week. Despite his busy work schedule, he plans for ninety minutes a day, half cardio and half weight training.

One day his assistant called my office in a panic. She explained that her employer needed to see me ASAP. When I asked the reason, she said, "His self-image is crumbling, and with it his edge in business. Help!"

Jason arrived on time, with a deep tan and dressed in a designer suit and tie, with Prada shoes and a flashy gold watch. He looked impeccable.

But he explained there was a chink in his perfect armor. Recently things had changed for reasons that perplexed him. Despite sticking to his mainly vegetarian diet, intensive workouts, meditation, and major vitamin regimen, something was happening around his middle.

His abs were hiding behind a distinct covering of fat, and his thirty-two-inch waist had recently increased to thirty-four inches—and his 34 jeans were getting tight.

As I looked at his food diary I saw a pattern. Although he avoided junk food, fast food, fatty meats, butter, creamy dressings, and dessert, his semivegetarian diet was *very* high in carbohydrate.

Breakfast: A fruit smoothie, sixteen ounces, made with *lots of fruit, agave nectar*, egg whites, and *fat-free fruited yogurt*

Lunch: Sautéed tofu, black beans, and veggies over *brown rice*, and a glass of *fresh-squeezed juice*

Late-afternoon gym: *Gatorade*™ throughout his high-intensity workout

Snack: A box of *raisins* and a *high-carb* protein shake

Dinner: Shrimp, *brown rice*, lentils, *whole-grain Indian bread*, and iced green tea sweetened with *honey*

On paper Jason was eating a reasonable number of calories and his intake was low in fat and high in fiber, vitamins, and antioxidants—technically it should not promote a bulging belly. I circled the carbohydrate foods and went on to look through Jason's recent lab work, highlighting the labs in the Met B range:

Glucose: 93 (Met B)
LDL cholesterol: 113 (Met B)
HDL cholesterol: 62 (normal)
Triglycerides 125 (Met B)
TSH: 2.6 (his thyroid was normal)
Vitamin D: 36 (Met B)

He told me that when his labs came back his doctor pronounced him in perfect health. I looked at the labs and pronounced him as Met B.

When I told Jason about Met B, he was fascinated—and hopeful. "I had never before heard of insulin imbalance, and maybe this is the missing link for me. I thought I was doing so well with my diet, exercise, and lifestyle."

Directly after our session he stopped at the grocery store and committed to starting MM the next morning.

Before our eight-week follow-up I received an e-mail from Jason. He wanted me to know he once again fit into his size 32 jeans, was beginning to see signs of his "six-pack," and felt like his old self. People remarked he was looking younger, more toned, and "oh so handsome." Jason was once again walking on sunshine.

That sounds fine, you say, for someone who has the luxury of dedicating so much time to his eating patterns and exercise regimen. But what about someone whose schedule makes flexibility impossible? What about someone who works full time and travels frequently?

No Time for This!

Cheryl, a fifty-six-year-old VP of marketing for a large corporation, had just received the phone call. She had type 2 diabetes.

She recently had her annual blood tests and left the lab feeling confident all was well. She returned to her life, not giving the labs a second thought. She was told she would hear from her physician only if he needed to discuss something. Although her father and paternal grandfather had type 2 diabetes and her brother had recently developed prediabetes, it never occurred to Cheryl that she might get this phone call. And now, ten days later, she sat shaking from the news.

A take-charge person, Cheryl looked for a certified diabetes educator to learn more about what she could do to "cure" her diabetes. "I don't have time for this," she told me. "I'm very busy, under tons of stress. I hate to cook—I'm always at business lunches and dinners and I travel most of the time. Please teach me what I need to know, and I'll beat this."

"I'll teach you to *control* this, Cheryl, but type 2 diabetes is not a curable disease."

"I read online that diabetes *can* be cured."

"You *can* control type 2 and live a long and very normal life, and I can help you stay far away from needing insulin or medications."

I learned Cheryl was a confirmed career person. She lived alone and was used to being able to come and go as she pleased. She was never fond of cooking, and even when she was home, she often picked up her lunch or dinner.

Cheryl stated she was five-foot-six inches and 187 pounds. She worked hard to conceal her excess weight. She had learned how to "dress thin" and stand tall. She wore heels, was a fan of Spanx™, and favored black and navy for her work attire.

When she stepped on my scale she was shocked to see she weighed 195 pounds. And when I checked her height, she had lost an inch and was now five-foot-five inches! "At my last annual physical exam I weighed 187 pounds, and the year before I was 182 pounds. What is happening to me?"

Cheryl learned that she did, indeed, have Met B, as she had a diagnosis of type 2 diabetes. In addition to her elevated blood glucose, she also had elevated total cholesterol, LDL, triglycerides, and low vitamin D and HDL cholesterol. Her bone density had also decreased. In short, Cheryl had the full complement of Metabolism B labs. And her lab work from two years ago showed the same thing.

But Cheryl was never alerted to her hypertension, elevated glucose showing prediabetes, lipids, or low vitamin D.

Cheryl was furious. If she had known her status, she would have taken action years ago.

I explained that it is very important to ask for your blood pressure readings when your pressure is checked and always get a copy of lab work. From now on she would keep track of her weight, measurements, glucose, A1C, lipid panel, TSH, and vitamin D level to look for trends.

We made a chart of her BP, height, weight, measurements, and labs. I told her that if she followed the program, the next time her labs were checked she could expect major improvements in every area.

When I showed Cheryl the MM lifestyle plan we discussed how to modify it based on her lifestyle, distaste for cooking, and frequent business travel. She was pleased to configure normal meals and snacks and learn how to order in a restaurant the MM way. We also discussed exercise and how she would manage to fulfill that MM requirement even with her long hours and travel.

When I next saw Cheryl she was happy to report she had lost eleven pounds of fat and twelve inches. She was thrilled that the fat loss from the MM program made her appear as if she had lost ten to fifteen more pounds than the scale showed. Her blood sugar log showed all normal readings, and they had normalized within five days of beginning the program. She did not need any medication for diabetes, blood pressure, or cholesterol, and her vitamin D was in the normal range. Another benefit? She had more energy, felt less anxious, and had more focus and concentration. And she looked *great* in her clothes.

This Is You

By now you probably realize your carbohydrate metabolism is different. You need never again try to force a square peg into a round hole because the Metabolism Miracle is a lifetime lifestyle plan that matches *your* metabolism. This program will help you lose weight, keep it off, and improve your emotional and physical well-being with as little medication as possible.

3

Understanding Your
Unique Metabolism

The Metabolism Miracle is not a typical low-carb diet. Other low-carb diets are written for the general public as a means to lose weight and, in some cases, decrease blood lipids.

People never seem to achieve permanent weight loss on standard low-carb diets unless they remain in the very low-carb stage and never move forward. Anyone with uncontrolled Met B who attempts to lose weight with a standard low-carb diet will regain what they lost as soon as they try to reintroduce even healthy carbs. When you reintroduce healthy, gentle carb grams on Step Two of MM, you will do so in a very methodical way, with attention paid to the amount, type, and timing of carbs so that fat burning and weight loss continues.

Unlike standard low-carb diets, the three steps of the Metabolism Miracle program are designed to *retrain* your body to process carbohydrate normally. Before you begin the program you should understand how your metabolism differs and causes you to struggle with weight and weight-related health conditions.

Imagine your weight as a fast-growing, out-of-control weed. If you try to destroy the weed by cutting it down with the lawn mower but leave the hidden root behind, the weed will survive and regrow. In the same way, if you simply treat your weight and weight-related medical conditions with diet restrictions and medications but never get to the root of the problem, your weight will continue to increase.

Uncontrolled Metabolism B causes your body to overreact to carbohydrate foods. The Met B pancreas overreacts to any increase in blood glucose by releasing *excess* insulin, a fat-storage hormone. Too much insulin causes excessive fat storage in both the blood, in the form of cholesterol and triglycerides, and the body, in the form of that roll of fat around your middle.

The roots of your weight and medical problems include:

- excessive insulin release in response to rising blood glucose
- increasing resistance to your body's own insulin
- excess glycogen release from the liver in response to a temporary drop in blood glucose

Once you destroy the root, the weed's offshoots—weight, cholesterol, hypertension, and blood glucose issues—will wither away and stay under control with little to no medication.

Although other diets may succeed for a short period of time, they don't maintain weight loss because they fail to address Met B's overreaction to a rise in blood glucose. The Metabolism Miracle is designed to get to the root and retrain your body to process carbohydrate and release glycogen stores in a normal way.

Knowing what is different about your body is half the battle; the other half is in learning how to manage your Met B metabolism. That's where the Metabolism Miracle program comes into play and teaches you to work with your body instead of against it.

A Bagel in the Life of Metabolisms A and B

To understand how Metabolism B reacts to carbohydrates, let's compare you with a friend who has Metabolism A.

You and your friend plan to take a hike. Early in the morning, on the way to the hiking trail, you decide to grab a bagel and coffee. You figure the bagel will give you lots of energy by "carb loading" your muscles before the long trek. You've got this, right? Wrong.

A bagel is a very dense carbohydrate food: one bagel can equal the carbohydrate grams of four to five slices of bread.

Carbohydrates convert into glucose (sugar) that is then released into the bloodstream. The brain detects the rapid rise in blood glucose and instructs the pancreas to release the right amount of insulin to help bring high blood glucose back into the normal range. When the bagel is processed, any glucose above the body's normal blood glucose (65 to 100 mg/dL) will refill glycogen stores in the muscles (the stores you use to move, exercise, and breathe) and liver (the stores you burn when others have been depleted). But after the muscles and liver are filled to their capacity, any remaining excess blood glucose will be stored as fat.

So blood glucose from the carbohydrate grams in the bagel needs to get inside the muscle cells and liver. Think of blood glucose as needing a "key" to "open the doors" of muscle, the liver, and fat cells. Insulin is the key that opens the cells' doors and enables glucose to leave the blood and enter the cells.

Your Met A friend's pancreas releases the exact number of insulin keys to return her blood glucose to the normal range, replenish the liver and muscle cells, and store any excess glucose in fat cells. After eating her bagel your friend feels full, energized, and ready to go. She will remain satisfied during the four to five hours this fueling process takes.

But your Met B pancreas over-releases insulin keys to deal with the bagel's glucose rush. Once the insulin helps refill glycogen stores in the muscles and liver, any excess insulin keys then open excess fat cells. The overabundance of insulin keys open too many fat cells and usher excess glucose from your bloodstream into the open fat cells. As glucose enters all the opened fat cells, blood glucose is depleted beyond the normal range. You are left with too little blood glucose to fuel your brain, supply normal energy, and provide the feeling of satiation or fullness. Your blood glucose has momentarily dipped below the normal range.

And so after eating the same bagel as your Met A friend, you end up fatter than she is. Your brain will sense the lower than normal blood glucose, causing you to begin to feel tired, washed out, and hungry. All these consequences occur within a few hours after eating. You look at your friend—she feels great with no fatigue or hunger. What a woman!

As you proceed with the hike you feel the urge to eat granola—now! Your brain is signaling you to find and eat carbohydrates, the one type of food that will *quickly* bring blood glucose up to normal. You start to feel a bit lightheaded, wiped out, empty, and irritable. Meanwhile your friend climbs the hiking trail, singing all the way.

THE BAGEL BOMB

Depending upon your metabolism, a bagel can cause two very different reactions in the body. This chart illustrates how the paths diverge.

You and your friend both eat a bagel.

↓

The bagel's carbohydrate turns to blood glucose and enters the bloodstream.

↓

The brain senses the blood glucose rise and instructs the pancreas to release the hormone insulin.

↙ ↘

Metabolism A *and the Bagel*

↓

The pancreas releases exactly the right amount of insulin to handle the rise in blood glucose.

↓

Insulin acts like a key and opens the right amount of fat and muscle cells and returns the glucose in the bloodstream to normal.

↓

Glucose from the bagel provides immediate energy, replaces glycogen in muscle and liver, and any excess is stored as fat.

↓

Equilibrium results in the body feeling satisfied and full after the meal.

↓

Satisfaction lasts for four to five hours until hunger naturally occurs.

Metabolism B *(YOU) and the Bagel*

↓

The pancreas overreacts and releases excess insulin to handle the rise in blood glucose.

↓

Excess insulin opens excess fat cells, ushers in the glucose and leaves too little glucose in the blood for basic energy. Your fat cells get microscopically larger and receptors "stretch" a bit.

↓

The brain signals you to eat more carbohydrate to quickly raise the blood glucose. You feel hungry, tired, shaky, nauseated, and irritable until you eat a carbohydrate snack.

↓

You temporarily feel better as blood glucose rises.

↓

Your brain senses a rise in blood glucose and tells the pancreas to once again release insulin.

↓

Your pancreas over-releases again and the cycle repeats itself.

If you cave and eat your honey-toasted granola bar, you will immediately feel better, but only for a short time. The carbohydrates contained in the granola will return your blood glucose to normal and temporarily boost your low blood sugar. You might even hear yourself thinking, *This is the best granola on earth!* Just as quickly, though, you admonish yourself for snacking again. You always find yourself having a meal and then snacking a few hours afterward.

Although you appear to be out of control, gobbling granola even as you desperately desire to lose weight, you are actually following your brain's direction as it seeks to bring your blood glucose into a normal range.

The satisfaction and euphoria you feel lasts a short time. When the granola digests and blood glucose begins to rise, your brain will once again call upon your Met B pancreas. Just like after the bagel, your Met B pancreas will respond with excess insulin. The cycle repeats itself as excess fat cells receive excess glucose, and your blood glucose levels dip into the low zone.

Behind the scenes you are slowly but surely becoming fatter. To add insult to injury, the insulin receptor sites (the keyholes) on the surface of your fat cells are gradually stretching, making it more difficult for your insulin keys to open the cells. You feel your energy level dropping once more, and again you will have the urge to eat.

When the hike is over you are embarrassed to ask your friend to stop immediately for lunch.

What if you simply ignore your brain and refuse to give in and eat? What if you remain steadfast and ignore your cravings? What if you take the long way home without eating lunch or a snack? Maybe you would be thinner if you just ignored the carbohydrate cravings. Surprisingly, the answer for people with Metabolism B is no.

The Beast Within

The human body has many built-in survival mechanisms, back-up systems that help keep you functioning and alive. A specific survival mechanism adds to the challenges people with uncontrolled Metabolism B face. This mechanism occurs in all people, Met A or Met B, but adds to weight issues for those with Met B. It is very seldom mentioned when discussing weight loss and improved health. However, not knowing about this mechanism is 50 percent of the problem that causes fat gain for those with Met B, as it impacts your weight and health as much as carbohydrates do.

When blood glucose drops to the low end of normal and you choose *not* to eat, your liver will naturally step up to the plate and fuel your body with its glycogen stores.

The body has a five-hour clock that runs continually, day and night. Each time you eat appreciable carbohydrate, your body will run on glucose from the carb you consumed for four to five hours. If, after the glucose from your carbohydrate intake digests and absorbs (four to five hours later), you choose not to eat, your brain will send a STAT message to your Met B pancreas to release a different hormone: *glucagon*.

Glucagon travels in the blood to the liver and signals your liver to release stored blood glucose called *glycogen*. This glycogen release will push blood glucose levels back into the normal range. Releases of liver glycogen keep your body running until you next eat—that's the survival mechanism part.

If you have ever gone to bed hungry and the next morning you wake up no longer hungry, you are feeling the effects of the self-feeding response. Similarly, if you work through lunch without eating, you might feel hungry for a little while, but when you don't eat, the hunger passes. Your liver takes care of you by releasing glycogen to raise your blood glucose and satisfy the brain.

When you and your friend decided to postpone lunch, you both passed the five-hour mark, and both your livers naturally released glycogen. But your Met A friend's pancreas released the right amount of insulin, whereas your Met B pancreas over-released insulin and ferried blood glucose into excess fat cells. The same over-insulin cycle that happens when a person with Met B eats carbohydrate happens when a person with Met B fails to eat within four to five hours and the liver steps up to the plate. In a sense, those with Met B are darned when they eat, and darned when they don't eat.

As a result of an inherited insulin over-response to rises in blood glucose from carbohydrates and glycogen release, a person with uncontrolled Met B will gradually develop an apple shape with midline paunch,

UNDERSTANDING INSULIN RESISTANCE . . .
AS IT ADVANCES THE PROGRESSION OF MET B

By now you are most likely realizing that your fluffy belly fat is forming from over-release of the fat gain hormone, insulin. Excess insulin is a defining issue for those with uncontrolled Metabolism B.

Unfortunately the story does not end there, as people with uncontrolled Metabolism B have another challenge as well.

Imagine that insulin is like a key that must fit perfectly into a keyhole to open a door and allow access inside. If the keyhole is misshapen, the insulin key will not fit and the lock will not open. With uncontrolled Met B, as fat cells grow in size, their keyholes, known as insulin receptors, stretch and change shape until insulin keys no longer fit the receptor (lock) on the cell door. This is called insulin resistance. The person with uncontrolled Met B has excess insulin, but over time fewer and fewer insulin keys fit cell receptors. The cells are resisting insulin.

Blood glucose remains stacked up in the bloodstream as lots of excess insulin fails to open cell doors. Insulin also builds up in the blood, as it is no longer functional. At this point the person with uncontrolled Met B simultaneously has excessive insulin *and* excessive blood glucose.

When the brain detects the higher than normal blood glucose in the blood, it resignals the pancreas to release even more insulin. The pancreas is forced to work harder and harder to produce insulin. You ate, your blood

love handles, back fat, or muffin-top. He will eventually face elevations in blood pressure and cholesterol and will feel wiped out, unfocused, fatigued, and miserable. He lives with bouts of low blood sugar that will eventually turn him into a "carboholic." No wonder his self-esteem has plummeted and he feels out of control and frustrated.

He hasn't gained weight because he's gorged on large meals of fatty foods and calories; he's gained weight and inches because his pancreas releases excess insulin that opens excess fat cells. Those fat cells are fed at the expense of his normal blood sugar, and low blood sugar depletes his energy level. Of course, he craves more food as a result! He hasn't caused these problems, but he *can* improve and even correct the situation. And glucose rose, insulin was over-released, but your cells remain "unfed" and you begin to feel tired, irritable, fatigued, and very hungry.

A person with Metabolism A has cell receptors that never change shape, no matter how fat or how thin he becomes. Regardless of the size of a Met A's fat cells, insulin will always perfectly fit the insulin receptors and will always open the cell to receive glucose. When a 350-pound man with Met A eats, his insulin is always released in the appropriate amount to match his blood glucose *and* his insulin receptors and insulin fit as perfectly as they did when he weighed 200 pounds. He reached this weight from overeating, taking in excess calories, and not burning them off with activity. Any low-calorie diet and exercise will work for him.

If the 350-pound man has uncontrolled Met B, his insulin has long been over-released in response to rising blood glucose from the carbohydrates he eats and the glycogen his liver releases. As he progressively gained weight from 200 to 350 pounds, his insulin increased, fat cells became overgrown, insulin receptors stretched, and over a period of time his pancreas began to work extra hard to come up with insulin to match his rising blood sugar.

If insulin resistance is left untreated, the fatigued pancreas can no longer release enough insulin, and the insulin it releases no longer fits all the receptors. Continuously facing locked doors, blood glucose backs up in the bloodstream. This is the beginning of type 2 diabetes and explains why it's so important to use the Metabolism Miracle to stop the progression of Met B before it leads to this irreversible health challenge.

so can you. The three steps of the Metabolism Miracle will help you control and stop the progression of Metabolism B.

Your physician may or may not have mentioned insulin resistance or may not have informed you that you have prediabetes. The longer you live with the uncontrolled Metabolism B, the more advanced your weight and weight-related health conditions will become. Most people with uncontrolled Met B know they weigh much more than they should, given the quantity of food they eat, and that they can't lose weight and keep it off. They are progressively feeling older, sicker, and more depressed and anxious. No one believes they *are* trying to lose weight. But until now people did not know or understand Metabolism A vs. Metabolism B.

When I read the bagel story in *The Metabolism Miracle* my mouth literally fell open—this was me! Someone out there actually gets it! I started the program on December 26, 2011, and never looked back! I lost a total of fifty pounds and have never felt healthier or stronger! There is a history of diabetes in my family that used to haunt me, and I always felt like I was on a runaway train with food that would inevitably lead to that. I no longer feel this way; instead, I feel in control and confident. And this newfound confidence has spilled over into other areas of my life!

—*Carole Johnston*

Trouble Triggers: A Guide to Deciphering When and Why Metabolism B Progressed

Until your Metabolism B progressed to the point that symptoms appeared, your body seemed to respond to food like everyone else's, and most reasonable low-calorie, low-fat diets worked for you. At some point, however, your metabolism changed. You were born with the genetic predisposition and always had the potential for excess insulin release, insulin resistance, and resultant overweight and glucose issues, but for a good part of your life you coasted along without a clue. Research indicates that the progression to uncontrolled Met B is spirited by the genetic propensity to Met B plus certain life stressors.

Triggers that may be responsible for the onset and progression of Metabolism B include:

1. *Hormonal changes.* Growth spurts, puberty, pregnancy, perimenopause, menopause, and aging all cause dramatic hormonal shifts in your body.
2. *Stress.* Stressful challenges involved with adolescence, the college years, entering the adult workforce, marriage, children, career, divorce, or death of a loved one may trigger the symptoms of Metabolism B.
3. *Illness and pain.* The flu, a virus, surgery, back injury, broken bones, childbirth, severe arthritis, fibromyalgia, lupus, cancer,

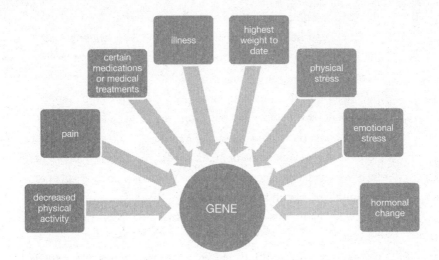

or a chronic illness can be the catalyst for Metabolism B's progression.

4. *Medications.* Certain medications for high blood pressure (beta blockers), antidepressants, and steroids such as cortisone and prednisone can cause the onset and progression of Met B symptoms.

5. *Excess weight.* The strain of excess body fat and increasing insulin resistance can push Met B's buttons.

6. *Physical inactivity.* Exercise helps to decrease blood sugar and insulin release.

The Timeline of Metabolism B

Now that you know of Metabolism B, it's helpful to look back over your life and assess when the symptoms for this alternate metabolism began to surface.

Put a check next to the time when your metabolism appeared to shift gears to Met B, and you'll find that from that point on, your weight issues, symptoms, temperament, and medical history began to change.

_____ Your birth weight was close to or over nine pounds.

_____ As a child you were either considered pencil thin or chubby. Your childhood pictures may not show you at a "normal" weight for height.

_____ Women may recall having their first menstrual period much earlier or much later than their friends. Some had severe PMS with irregular and heavy periods with clots and bad cramps.

_____ Despite being pencil thin or chubby as a child, your weight began to increase during your teens or midtwenties. You could no longer get away with dietary indiscretions and could gain five pounds in one weekend! You began to notice that even though you ate the same or less than your normal-weight friends, you were becoming heavier than they.

_____ You may have had difficulty getting pregnant and may have experienced one or more miscarriages. After pregnancy many women with Metabolism B report extreme frustration in their effort to lose the baby weight. After each delivery weight loss became even more difficult.

_____ Women who haven't had children may notice a change in their weight irrespective of childbirth. Their lifestyles may include feeling rushed and stressed with less time to exercise and relax.

_____ Men may notice that they begin to develop a midline paunch and a layer of fat over their abdominal area. They may develop love handles and a belly. Eventually they have difficulty buttoning their dress shirt at the neck and belly area. Their waistline has increased and continues to be a problem even if they get regular exercise. Work and family obligations may take precedence over gym time.

_____ Eventually weight-loss methods that successfully knocked off five or ten pounds in the past stop working. The older you are, the harder it becomes to lose weight. At some point you seemed to lose the battle and simply gave up hope.

_____ No matter what diet program you tried, your excess weight never came off and stayed off. Your friends made diet changes and got results; you made the same changes and gained weight!

_____ Your overall health began to change, and you needed medication for weight-related health problems. You decided to buy a pill box!

_____ You began to feel much older than your age. Your face looked puffy, and there were bags under your eyes. Your skin and hair lacked glow and shine. Your nails would not grow without splitting. You felt bloated, especially after eating a meal, and you needed to unbutton your jeans to breathe. You began to feel a variety of aches and pains and you felt tapped of energy. Mild depression and bouts of anxiety entered your life. You slept fitfully and woke up tired. You were uncomfortable in your body.

_____ Women's symptoms of perimenopause and menopause were magnified, and many *really* suffered with night sweats, mood swings, hot flashes, food cravings, depression, and crankiness. Your leaner friends seemed to have symptoms to a much lesser degree.

_____ Your carbohydrate addiction got worse. You opened the kitchen cabinets and went from bag to carton, bingeing on carb foods. After opening a bag of chips or cookies, you kept returning for more than you intended. You began to worry that you had lost all control. Why did you lack willpower?

Putting a check at the time you boarded the Met B train helps to put your present weight into perspective. Some have been battling the symptoms of Met B since they were children; others become symptomatic in their early adulthood or even middle age.

Debbie Demands Liposuction

Debbie M., a thirty-eight-year-old woman who was "through having babies," as she told me, grabbed her roll of belly fat and sighed, "I'm going to have liposuction and suck this darn roll off my body once and for all. None of my past diets work, I'm getting fatter, and my waistline has increased by four inches. I am more than twenty-five pounds heavier than before my pregnancies, and enough is enough." Debbie was now five-foot-five and weighed 175 pounds.

Since most of her fat was concentrated around her middle, liposuction seemed the perfect answer. She felt she would lose weight and her burgeoning waistline at the same time.

Plastic surgeons advise their patients to get as close as possible to their desired weight before the procedure because after most liposuctions, about five to seven pounds of tissue is removed. What is collected in the postsurgery container is not all fat; it also contains body fluids and

SOME COMMON FOOD EXPERIENCES OF THOSE WITH
UNCONTROLLED METABOLISM B

Over the years I've met with thousands of people with Metabolism B. To this day it amazes me to see the similarities in their experiences with food. Take a minute and see if you recognize yourself in the following commonalities.

- When dieting, the decreased quantity of food consumed does not reflect in lost weight. Family, friends, physicians, and nutritionists have assumed you are underreporting what you eat, are a closet eater or food binger, have bulimia, or simply lie on your food diary.
- People with Metabolism B have a history of yo-yo dieting and can recall losing and regaining hundreds of pounds throughout their lifetime. They feel frustrated, ashamed, confused, and despondent.
- The breakfast bomb: half of these patients aren't hungry in the morning and "cannot possibly" eat breakfast. The other half cannot function without eating as soon as they awaken in the morning. It's all or nothing regarding the first meal of the day! Whereas half of Met Bs skip breakfast, the other half choose a carbohydrate-heavy meal with some combination of toast, bagels, bars, fruit juice, cereal, Danish, muffins, doughnuts, fruit smoothies, or fruited yogurt.
- They feel they are in "their best control" before they eat anything for the day. They report feeling increasingly hungry once they begin to eat.
- Metabolism B patients often report needing to eat again within a few hours after a meal. Midmorning, late afternoon, and nighttime cravings and snacking are common. When they try to control themselves and hold off on eating, they get cranky, nauseated, irritable, weak, or lightheaded.
- After lunch, people with Metabolism B frequently feel drowsy and could use a nap. If they can't nap, they often report needing chocolate, a salty/crunchy snack, or caffeine in the afternoon. Most Met Bs relate needing a caffeine "lift" in the morning and late afternoon. They drink coffee, tea, iced tea, caffeinated soft drinks, or energy drinks or eat chocolate to boost their energy.
- Although they'd like to prepare a balanced dinner, these individuals list demanding careers, dual-career families, single-parent families, family commitments, and fatigue among the reasons they dine out or bring in dinner. Many report having pizza, Chinese take-out, deli food, fast food,

restaurant food, or take-out dinners several times a week, all of which are very high in carb grams.

- When eating out, most Met Bs try to ignore the bread basket, but once they begin sampling it, they have a difficult time controlling their consumption of bread and rolls.
- Most don't eat dessert as part of dinner (they are always trying to cut calories) but seem to have an overwhelming craving for sweets or salty, crunchy foods in the course of the evening. Ice cream or chips are favorite nighttime snacks.
- Pasta can cause a major problem for those with Metabolism B. Most admit to eating one or more full plates at the meal, snitching some as they clear the table, picking at the pasta in the refrigerator throughout the evening, and even digging into the pasta bowl in the morning.
- Many people with Metabolism B feel fixated on food, daydreaming about it throughout their day and even thinking about what they are going to eat for dinner as they eat their breakfast.
- Many report sleepiness after eating their nighttime meal and falling asleep in a chair as they watch the evening news. They wake up a little later in the evening, feeling empty and having a strong urge for nighttime snacking.
- A significant number wake up hungry in the middle of the night. Some get out of bed and head to the refrigerator at 2:00 or 3:00 a.m. for a snack. Others wake up and can't fall back asleep.

Almost every Metabolism B person I counsel reports eating more when he or she is under stress. People with Met A may have no appetite when they are going through a stressful period in their life. Met Bs typically can't stop snacking when they are stressed. Why? Stress normally raises blood sugar, and for those with Met B, that means lots of insulin release, low blood sugar, and carb cravings around the clock.

Interestingly, when your Metabolism B is finally controlled, the eating patterns that had been your way of life lessen or even disappear. People cannot believe the food choices they once craved and looked forward to eating no longer had that effect on them. It turns out the food wasn't really that delicious; it just provided the necessary blood glucose boost and literally gave comfort. When blood glucose stays in the normal zone, without peaks and valleys, carbohydrates become like any other food.

I was *always* a chubby kid. There was never a time in my life when I felt like it was fair—I truly *didn't* eat more than other people. In my midtwenties I recognized that type 2 diabetes, obesity, thyroid disease, cancer, and heart disease ran rampant in my family. I felt like a ticking time bomb, waiting for the day when weight and disease would overtake me. The Metabolism Miracle was going to be my last-ditch effort to lose weight before considering bariatric surgery. A year and a half into this program *I've lost sixty-eight pounds and dropped ten pant sizes.* The Metabolism Miracle saved my health and saved my life.

—*Barbara K.*

other components. In truth, a person usually loses two to three pounds of actual fat during the procedure.

Debbie realized she would only lose about six pounds on the scale, less than half of that would represent fat loss, and the fat that was removed would return somewhere else within a year. She also learned that the only fat that can be liposuctioned was directly under the skin. The fat between her organs could not be removed, as it is deep in her abdominal cavity under a layer of muscle. This deep fat between organs is associated with heart disease and diabetes. Research has shown that part of the fat that eventually returns after liposuction is deposited deep inside the belly, between and on the organs.

Debbie realized this procedure was not the answer for her. How could she lose inches and resculpt her body without liposuction's very temporary treatment and potentially unhealthy surgery?

That's when I began to explain Metabolism B and the Metabolism Miracle.

Liposuction and Those with Met B

A person is born with a certain number of fat cells. This number can change during childhood and adolescence, but after adolescence the number of fat cells remains very stable for the rest of your life. If you get fatter, you do not acquire more fat cells; the fat cells you already have get larger in size. When you lose weight the fat cells shrink. But the number remains constant.

Liposuction is a procedure in which fat is sucked and removed from specific areas of the body, and patients can see the fat that is removed after it is sucked into a container.

According to Robert H. Eckel, MD, professor of medicine at the University of Colorado, in an April 2011 study published in *Obesity,* "Liposuction can help sculpt and contour problem areas of the body, but the fat cells will be back within one year of surgery. When the fat returns, it will come back in different places like the upper abdomen, upper thighs, neck, back, and even the arms." Eckel believes the fat does not return to the previously liposuctioned area because the prior procedure damages the matrix of that tissue. But know this: the fat will return to your body's normal.[1]

The body will always maintain the number of fat cells you had after adolescence.

4

What Happened? Other Diets Used to Work for Me

By now you can understand how Met B causes your body to store excess blood glucose in an excessive number of fat cells.

The Metabolism Miracle will help you temper your pancreas, calm insulin release, decrease fat production so permanent weight loss can finally happen. But why wouldn't any diet help you lose weight?

When your friends with Metabolism A want to lose weight, they can follow any reasonable diet because their metabolism follows the classic formula found in any basic nutrition textbook:

$$\text{Calories eaten} - \text{calories burned} = \text{weight}$$

In other words, your friends who have Metabolism A will gain weight if they consume more calories than they burn off. They will lose weight if they cut back on total calories while increasing their physical activity. Your friends' cholesterol is determined by their weight, physical activity, and fatty food intake. Their triglycerides may increase because of excess alcohol or certain medications, and their blood pressure may increase from excess weight or sensitivity to sodium.

In contrast, the Met B's weight, body fat, cholesterol, triglycerides, blood pressure, and blood sugar are linked to insulin imbalance and excess fat stores.

You now know your metabolism is very different. The law of calories doesn't apply to people with Metabolism B. You may eat far fewer calories than your friends and might even lose weight initially. But your body makes excess insulin and stores excess blood glucose as fat. A diet based on calories will never work for you in the long term. Your weight, midline fat, and cholesterol are not entirely the result of excess calories or inadequate physical activity; they are caused by the hyper-metabolism of carbohydrate and excess blood glucose being stored in fat cells. You are a fat producer as long as your Met B remains uncontrolled.

Help Me, Doc

Most people with Metabolism B have been told by their physician, "You need to lose twenty pounds—or even more." Naturally you are very aware that you need to lose twenty pounds, but despite all of your attempts, you can't seem to make it happen. If you have hypertension, you hear, "Cut down on salt and lose some weight." When your cholesterol rises, you hear, "Reduce fats and lose some weight." If you progress to diabetes, the advice changes only slightly: "Watch your sugar intake and lose some weight." Unfortunately that's the extent of the nutrition advice many patients hear. They leave their doctor's office with a handful of prescriptions, a diet sheet, and a follow-up appointment date. The doctor has not given people with Metabolism B the key to successful weight loss.

In an effort to find some answers some patients seek out a registered dietitian (RD) and leave that appointment with a copy of the same fifteen-hundred-calorie, low-fat/low-cholesterol/low-salt playbook the RD uses for everyone in your condition. But all the hard work and effort these patients put into following the calorie-based guidelines they received from their healthcare team will be in vain if they have Met B. If you have Metabolism B, this standard diet, based on "calories in" minus "calories out," will never work for you.

Misguided Guidelines

The medical community has known about metabolic syndrome, or Syndrome X (Metabolism B), for over fifty years. They have long been aware that certain people gradually develop a compilation of medical

THE NATIONAL INSTITUTES OF HEALTH: SOME PEOPLE HAVE DIFFICULTY LOSING WEIGHT BECAUSE OF DIFFERENCES IN METABOLISM

The medical community's advice has always been: in order to lose weight you must decrease calories and increase physical activity. We can clearly see what happens when a person with Metabolism B uses a traditional weight-loss diet: the further along the progression of Met B, the more difficult it is for dieters to lose weight and keep it off and get healthy. Although we annually spend billions on weight loss, we also face epidemic levels of obesity, diabetes, and weight-related medical conditions.

Researchers at the National Institutes of Health (NIH) recently published "scientific proof" supporting the belief that "people with certain physiologies lose less weight than others when limiting calories." They referred to people who lose less weight as having a "thrifty metabolism." Although NIH's study group was *very* small—just twelve participants—they labeled the results of this twelve-person study as "scientific proof."[1]

What NIH's study calls a "thrifty metabolism" is what I call uncontrolled Metabolism B. In my practice less than 40 percent of people succeed in losing weight on low-calorie-based diets, whereas 60 percent require a carbohydrate-balancing program.

The NIH researchers stated, "While behavioral factors such as adherence to diet affect weight loss to an extent, our study suggests we should consider a larger picture that includes individual physiology—and that weight loss is one situation where being 'thrifty' doesn't pay."

"What we've learned from this study may one day enable a more personalized approach to help people who are obese achieve a healthy weight," said Director Griffin P. Rodgers, MD.

Let's start now! For those with uncontrolled Met B (excess insulin production, insulin resistance, and fat gain), the lifestyle and diet solution is the Metabolism Miracle program.

conditions (a syndrome) that contributes to excess weight/obesity, elevated cholesterol and triglycerides, hypertension, and higher than normal blood sugar.

At the discovery of metabolic syndrome, medical advisers made a decision on the type of diet to recommend for those with this insulin-related syndrome.

Instead of recommending a carb-controlled diet with methodical re-introduction of lower glycemic carbohydrates, the scientists chose the low-fat, low-cholesterol, "calories in–calories out" approach. The assumption was that by lowering fat and cholesterol intake, it should follow that people would lose weight and excess body fat as well as lower their cholesterol and blood pressure.

History now shows that this diet did not curtail heart and blood vessel disease. In fact, over those fifty years people became fatter and sicker as they focused on a low-fat, low-cholesterol, and low-calorie lifestyle. No one seemed to notice that these diet recommendations forced a diet that was higher in carbohydrates. Over 60 percent of adults struggling with weight loss have major issues metabolizing carbohydrates. Over their lifetimes the low-fat, low-cholesterol, low-calorie diet (i.e., a high-carb diet) would work against them.

Although hundreds of books have been written to address the specific symptoms and medical conditions of uncontrolled Met B, diets for insulin resistance or metabolic syndrome do not cover all the underpinnings of Met B that progress to metabolic syndrome, prediabetes, being overweight, obesity, and type 2 diabetes.

The Metabolism Miracle differs from every other weight-loss book, as it is designed to cover *all* the facets of the Met B metabolism.

The medical associations responsible for setting diet guidelines have never developed or put their seal of approval on an effective diet and lifestyle plan for the population with Metabolism B. Unfortunately the older and current diet guidelines can harm a person with uncontrolled Met B. Metabolism B is progressive, and the longer it remains uncontrolled, the more damage it causes.

Please understand that traditional diet guidelines were written as if everyone processed food in the same way and were considered the gold standard before insulin imbalance/insulin resistance was formally identified. Unfortunately, even with the knowledge of metabolic syndrome, Syndrome X, or Metabolism B, diet recommendations have stayed the same.

As a registered dietitian, I originally used those medically sanctioned guidelines. This is what registered dietitians were instructed to teach, the gold standard for weight loss. After fifteen years working within these guidelines I felt compelled to research and develop the Metabolism Miracle.

Now that we understand that uncontrolled Metabolism B progresses to insulin imbalance and insulin resistance, metabolic syndrome, prediabetes, and type 2 diabetes, it's astounding how misguided most of the medical establishment's guidelines continue to be.

This type of carbohydrate-dense diet logic would make sense if everyone had Metabolism A. But we now know that a large portion of the population, including the majority of people with diabetes and heart disease, has Metabolism B. No wonder patients with heart disease who follow low-fat/low-cholesterol diets can rarely get their lipids to normalize and must instead depend on taking statins and other medications to control hypertension and cholesterol.

Recommending that those who have trouble processing carbohydrate should consume more than half of their calories from carbohydrate is like advising people with a milk allergy to consume half of their daily calories from dairy foods!

The "Carb Is a Carb" Myth

Perhaps you've heard the mantra, "A carb is a carb." This is the basis for yet another dietary myth: a carb is a carb because every gram of consumed carbohydrate will ultimately become blood glucose.

After this precedent, RDs began to teach patients that there was no difference between types of carbohydrate: thirty grams of carbohydrate from either sugar-sweetened yogurt or plain yogurt, fresh fruit or fruit juice, white flour or whole grain flour, desserts, regular soda, or legumes are all the same because the number of carb grams is the same. This carb-counting theory mesmerized my patients who had diabetes. By the carb-counting method, choosing a donut over whole-grain rice should have the same impact on their blood glucose. With carb gram counting, there was no longer a need to avoid dessert, juice, or candy as long as the carb grams equaled their recommended grams of carb per meal or snack.

To illustrate the "carb is a carb" theory, consider that both one slice of whole-wheat toast and a half a cup of orange juice contain about fifteen grams of carbohydrate each. Carbohydrate counting suggests choosing carbohydrates in the same number of grams from *any food* category: fruit, milk, starch, sugar, juice, grains, starchy veggies, or sweets will cause blood glucose to rise equally.

The problem with the original carbohydrate counting is that different food sources of carbohydrate change into blood glucose at different speeds and with different intensities.

When you drink half a cup of juice, your blood glucose will immediately increase with a sharp spike. By contrast, the whole-wheat toast or any carbohydrate that is naturally higher in fiber and lower in sugar grams will change to blood glucose at a slower speed without the intense spike.

Lower-impact carbohydrates, such as brown rice or whole-grain bread, have more staying power; they do not cause the pancreas to release a quick flood of insulin. Instead, their slower change into blood glucose prompts a slower release of insulin. In the medical world a carbohydrate's impact on blood glucose is determined by its *glycemic index,* which rates how rapidly a particular carbohydrate food turns into glucose. With the Metabolism Miracle, with an understanding that not all carbohydrate types are created equally, carb choices are categorized as *low impact (mild carbs)* and *high impact (wild carbs).*

You can see how the "carb is a carb" myth becomes a problem. When someone with Metabolism B chooses high-impact carbs, such as white potatoes or white rice, they tax their insulin response much more than if they were to eat exactly the same number of carbohydrate grams but in a low-impact form, such as sweet potatoes or brown rice. The fiber in whole grains enables them to have a "timed release" impact on blood glucose. (Adding fiber to a high-impact food does *not* change its glycemic index, as the carb grams inherent in the food will still have their high impact.)

THE WAKE-UP CALL

Sometimes people who look like the picture of health have a frightening wake-up call. That's when knowing that they have Metabolism B becomes a matter of life or death.

Anthony loved his active lifestyle. He really did look like the picture of health; the way he took care of his body obviously agreed with him. He had been married for over thirty years, recently cut down his work load to decrease stress, and finally had more spare time to spend golfing. The fifty-five-year-old was looking forward to retirement, when he would golf more.

He adhered to the diet and lifestyle changes his physician recommended years ago. At that time he had put on a few extra pounds around the middle and his blood pressure and cholesterol had begun to creep up. He faithfully took his statin and blood pressure medication, walked on the golf course, and stuck to his low-fat, low-cholesterol diet regimen. His friends and family chuckled as he ordered the leanest cut of beef, removed the skin from his chicken, used vinegar as his salad dressing, and skipped the butter on his dinner roll (or rolls!). His snacks included fat-free pretzels, fresh fruit with fat-free whipped cream, reduced-fat or fat-free ice cream, fat-free yogurt, and even fat-free cookies. He was determined to do as he was told to live a long, healthy, energetic life. He joked that when he was ninety-nine years of age, he wanted to die on the golf course—playing his favorite game.

He was shocked when, at the age of fifty-five, his friends called 911 in the middle of their golf outing. An hour later, in CCU, Anthony was told he had had a heart attack.

No one expected cardiac problems in a man who was so careful, so cautious, and so health conscious.

A few weeks after his heart attack Anthony sat across from me at my desk. He was angry and confused. "I did everything I was told to do—everything," he told me. "How could I possibly have a heart attack?"

I listened to Anthony's story and took a good look at the man who had followed traditional diet guidelines to the letter. He had a small roll of fat around his middle despite daily exercise and his strict low-fat, low-choles-terol diet. He complained of afternoon fatigue and feeling very sleepy after dinner, but he had a hard time falling and staying asleep.

He admitted that although he loved his wife and enjoyed her company, his libido had tanked, and Anthony had recently visited his MD for "the little blue pill."

His father had died of a heart attack at the age of sixty, and his own lab report was telling, with a fasting glucose of 112 (normal is 65 to 99 mg/dL [3.6 to 5.5 mmol/L]), and despite his medication, exercise, and diet, his LDL cholesterol, triglycerides, and blood pressure were all slightly higher than normal. In fact, his fasting glucose showed he was now prediabetic. But his doctor had always told him he was doing great and never mentioned the higher-than-normal lab work. He was shocked to learn that he still had less-than-healthy lab work.

I explained that a low-fat/low-cholesterol diet is high in carbohydrate and was probably partly responsible for moving his Metabolism B down the tracks as it over-processed blood glucose into fat. The diet he had so faithfully followed was working against him and may even have been a con-tributing factor to his prediabetes and heart attack.

Anthony was so entrenched in his low-fat/low-cholesterol diet mindset that he found it very difficult to transition to a different way of eating. Fortu-nately lean protein choices, heart-healthy fats, and lots of neutral veggies are a perfect backdrop for the Metabolism Miracle program, but he had to make major adjustments regarding his carbohydrate intake. Anthony was desperate and wanted his health back—yesterday.

Eight weeks after he began the Metabolism Miracle Anthony returned to my office, having lost four inches of fat off his belly. His blood pressure had normalized, and his medication for hypertension had already been de-creased. He felt energetic and confident and was thrilled with the ease of the program. He smiled as he told me that right after our meeting he was headed to the golf course.

When you have Metabolism B you must toss out the old carbohydrate and calorie myths to achieve permanent weight loss and avoid health issues down the road. It took me a long time to figure out how to save myself from the black hole of textbook diets, but like my patients who have followed the Metabolism Miracle program, I have normalized my weight, improved my health and well-being, and have gained boundless energy.

MM Is Not a Low-Carb Diet!

The Metabolism Miracle is not another low-carb diet. Unfortunately the program gets lumped into the same category as low-carb diets like Paleo, Atkins™, Dukan™, and South Beach™.

The Metabolism Miracle is a three-step lifetime lifestyle program, not a temporary diet. Step One is a lower carb phase, but it is only the beginning of the program. And even MM's first step allows many neutral foods and five grams of Counter Carbs that are not part of other low-carb diets.

Diets are for the short term. People may begin a diet to lose weight before an upcoming event like a wedding, vacation, or class reunion. When they reach the size they want to be, their diet is over. Those with uncontrolled Met B who are following a "diet" can lose eight to ten pounds—mainly muscle and water weight—but will stop losing and begin regaining when their insulin over-release, insulin resistance, and fat gain sets in.

It's so important to understand that Metabolism B is not curable; it is the result of a compilation of genes and lifestyle stressors that leave many people with uncontrolled insulin release and insulin resistance. Met B is controllable, but *you* are responsible for its control. If you pass through the steps of MM and reach your desired weight with great health and energy, you have controlled Met B. If you return to eating or avoiding carbs in a haphazard way, you will once again revert to uncontrolled Met B.

As a person with Met B, you need to learn to live *with* your metabolism. Eating lots of carbohydrate foods, skipping meals or snacks, doing cleanses, fasting, even overeating all healthy carbs is living *outside* the rules of your metabolism. It simply won't work for you.

So start off knowing that MM can eventually become your lifestyle. You will find yourself making the right choices with little or no thought.

When you reach your desired size, feel your best, look your best, and take as little medication as possible, you will move to maintenance on MM's Step Three.

PART TWO

The Three-Step Plan to Lose Weight and Get Your Health and Energy Back

5

Step One—Carb Detox

Eight Weeks to a Better Life

Think of Step One as cleaning up a messy, cluttered house. Clothes on the floor, piles of laundry, dirty windows, unkempt bathrooms, dusty floors and furniture, and papers strewn about make this home an uncomfortable place to live.

When you begin to clean up the house you accept it will take time, energy, focus, and effort. It will not be ship-shape in a day or two. It took a long time to get into a state of disarray, and it will take a while to get back to clean and orderly. Once it's back to normal you will function better in the house, and it will be a joy to return home after a day's work. Once you get the house under control it will be so much easier to keep it that way.

Your metabolic mess took a long time to get to this point, and it has long taken control of your daily life. It will take time and effort to turn this ship around, but once your metabolism is rested and reprogrammed, it will return to its original state. What's more, it will be much easier to keep it that way.

During Step One you will temporarily eliminate dense carbohydrate grams but can enjoy liberal quantities of lean protein, healthy fat, and neutral veggies.

This step will give your pancreas and liver a long-overdue vacation so they can rest and then reprogram to handle carbohydrates normally. By temporarily eliminating dense-carb foods, your blood glucose will automatically decrease and require less insulin from the pancreas. After day five of Step One's clean-up your liver will have temporarily lost most of its glycogen stores and will contribute less glucose between meals and during sleep. You should feel no cravings, be in control of what you eat, sleep better, and start burning fat. As you normalize your Met B metabolism, you will eventually create a clean slate on which to reintroduce carbs. You are setting the stage for a future at the size you desire and feeling younger, healthier, and more energetic.

Before I researched metabolic syndrome and developed the program I was not a fan of low-carb diets. I could not see a benefit from practically eliminating an entire food group. Carbohydrate is the preferred fuel for the body and mind, so how could *temporarily* eliminating dense carbs be healthy?

After years of researching Metabolism B I changed my mind. As it turns out, there is a way to nonmedicinally control the blood glucose and insulin imbalance that plagues people with this alternate metabolism. The program would *temporarily* eliminate most dense carbohydrates from the diet. This rehabilitative state helps accomplish two things:

1. Temporarily eliminating carb-dense foods enables a normalization of blood glucose and insulin release.
2. After less than one week on Step One of the Metabolism Miracle the liver will release most of its glycogen stores contributing to blood glucose during the self-feeding mechanism.

The body can handle a small amount of carbohydrate in protein, fat, and neutral veggies and still get a rest from the metabolic mess.

For the duration of Step One your blood glucose will run smoothly without high spikes that stimulate the pancreas to over-release insulin. Your pancreas and liver will temporarily take a much-needed vacation to rest and rejuvenate.

A low-carb diet is not nutritionally sound, but as a *temporary* method to reset an uncontrolled Met B metabolism, it does the job by deliberately leaving the pancreas and liver in a state of rest and rehab. Dense carbs will return in Steps Two and Three, but by then you have established normal blood glucose and insulin balance in your body.

The Five-Day Kicker

By the fifth day of Step One you will begin to notice a difference in the way you feel. A clearer mind, more stable mood, the beginning of better sleep, and a return of your energy are no small matters. But the first five days of Step One can be tough—the very reason I've nicknamed Step One "Detox."

Since the day you were born your body and mind have utilized the glucose from carbohydrates and glycogen release as their major fuel source. Because of your genetic predisposition to insulin imbalance after a series of life stressors, you began to overprocess carbohydrates. Your body is in a state of metabolic chaos, and it will take a few days for your body to acclimate to Step One.

For the first five days you may feel tired, cranky, hungry (even as you eat plenty of noncarb food), carb-crazy, slightly shaky, lightheaded, and a little headachy. Hold on—*you can do this.*

After five days you will begin to feel much better, with more energy and no carb cravings. You will also be less irritable and much more relaxed. Within a week, when Step One is in full swing, you will have no carb cravings, and your friends and family will probably mention how pleasant you are to be around and how much better you look.

Why can those first five days be difficult? Your liver contains approximately three days of blood glucose in the form of stored glycogen. When

WHAT IF I HAVE NO SYMPTOMS DURING THE FIRST FIVE DAYS OF MM? AM I DOING SOMETHING WRONG?

There are some people who report no "off" symptoms during their first five days of the program. Some of these dieters began the program with close-to-normal glucose and lipid levels and had not been overdosing on carbohydrate foods prior to starting Step One. Their "norm" is not much different from MM's Step One, so they don't feel the sharp peaks and valleys of a person whose Met B is further off track. If you have no symptoms when you begin Step One, you are one of the fortunate ones! It's not necessary to feel poorly the first days of the program, and those who have no symptoms will still lose within their expected fat/inch loss.

you begin Step One and temporarily eliminate dense carbohydrate grams from your diet, your liver will be thrust into the self-feed mode, providing a meal's worth of glycogen around the clock in four- to five-hour glycogen releases. In response to each of those self-fed meals, your Met B pancreas will continue to over-release insulin, and your blood sugar will continue to roller-coaster even though you will not be eating appreciable carbohydrate. Those blood sugar spikes and lows from glycogen release will initially make you irritable and cranky. Hold tight until the ride is over.

Ten Easy Guidelines: Rules to Thrive By

At the end of Step One's first five days, as you continue to eliminate dense carbohydrates and your liver and muscles are depleted of most of their glycogen stores, your brain will have to come up with an alternative plan for fueling the body. As long as you continue to eliminate dense carbs and your liver remains largely depleted of glycogen, the brain will choose between consuming muscle or fat for the body's energy needs.

This is why exercise is 50 percent of the Metabolism Miracle lifestyle. Physical activity literally ignites, energizes, and activates muscle tissue. The brain will always choose to burn metabolically *inactive* fat tissue and bypass activated muscle tissue.

Step One resets your metabolism to work normally. It retains active muscle tissue for increased metabolic rate and a leaner, more toned body. It preferentially melts away belly and back fat. As fat is burned, cholesterol and triglycerides are also decreased. Step One stabilizes and normalizes your metabolism as it allows the body to adjust to more stable blood glucose and decreased insulin release. It also blocks the liver from over-releasing glycogen stores. Instead of overbuilding fat on your body and in your blood, Step One is a fat-burning facilitator.

To maximize your success and keep yourself in tip-top health, it is important that you follow ten easy guidelines while on the program. Once you weave these rules into the fiber of your lifestyle and enjoy the difference they make, you'll understand why I call them Rules to Thrive By. See Chapter 8 for more on these guidelines.

1. *Drink at least sixty-four ounces of water and/or caffeine-free fluids daily.*
2. *Avoid gaps of more than five hours without a meal or snack.* Spread your food intake throughout the entire day and even into the night. Within one hour of waking up and one hour before bed be sure to have a meal or snack.
3. *Take the recommended vitamins, minerals, and supplements,* especially during Step One, when you are eliminating dense carbs and the nutrients they contain. Always report supplements along with medications to your MD.
4. *Choose nonnutritive sweeteners with care.* I suggest the use of sucralose, stevia, or erythritol as sugar replacements. Please avoid aspartame, NutraSweet™, Equal™, or saccharin.
5. *Judge the carbohydrate content of packaged foods by reading the Nutrition Facts* and ingredients section of food labels and using "the MM formula." (See the simple formula on page 64.)
6. *Consider drinking two cups of green tea daily.* Avoid if you take blood thinners like Coumadin or Warfarin. Get MD approval for green tea, a natural blood thinner.
7. *Increase your physical activity* to include a minimum of thirty minutes, five times per week over and above your usual physical activity. (Chapter 9 has more on exercise.) Make it a habit to change up your exercise every four to eight weeks.

8. *Consume neutral foods liberally but not to excess.*
9. *Try to relax.* Take a few minutes each day to close your eyes, breathe deeply, shed your stress, and clear your mind. Get adequate rest. I recommend seven to nine hours of sleep per night.
10. *Make it a habit to think positively!* First thing in the morning and the last thing at night, remind yourself of your good health, weight loss, high energy level, continuing progress, and positive future.

Simple, Simple, Simple

Perhaps the best part about Step One, besides the fat loss and energy boost, is its ease and simplicity. During Step One all foods fall into one of two categories: yes or no. People find these food choices incredibly easy to make. You will be able to cook, eat out, and celebrate while staying on program.

Look at the Arrow Sheet in this chapter. Each of the four arrows represents a category of foods: dense carbohydrates (to avoid for now), lean protein, healthy fat, and neutral vegetables. During your eight or more weeks of Step One you may eat liberally from the lean protein, healthy fat, and neutral vegetable arrows, but avoid full servings of the foods in the dense carbohydrate arrow. You won't need to read food labels for the carb content contained in most neutral foods like nuts, cheese, tofu, or broccoli; only the dense carb-containing foods that are in the dense carb arrow or in the 5-gram Counter Carb space require a label check.

Consider posting a copy of the Arrow Sheet on your refrigerator or keeping one at the office or in your bag to remind you of the foods to avoid on Step One and those you may eat freely. You can find a copy of the Arrow Sheet at www.themetabolismmiracle.com, and there is an Arrow Sheet in this book (pages 60–61).

Although most foods contain a combination of nutrients, they are classified into their arrow by the main nutrient they contain. For example, flank steak, tuna, and chicken fit into the protein arrow; olive oil, salad dressing, mayo, and nuts fit into the fat arrow; and potatoes, fruit, pasta, bread, and yogurt fit into the dense carbohydrate arrow.

Sometimes a food group can be split into two different arrows. Let's use dairy foods as an example. Some foods in the dairy group, like milk and yogurt, are in the dense carbohydrate arrow, whereas cheese is in the protein arrow and butter is in the fat arrow. This is because milk and yogurt contain more carb grams, cheese contains more protein grams, and butter contains more fat grams. Milk impacts the blood glucose; cheese and butter do not.

Many people are surprised to learn that milk, fruit, whole grains, and dried beans/legumes fit into the dense carbohydrate arrow. Foods in the dense carb arrow significantly impact blood sugar and cause your uncontrolled Met B pancreas to over-release insulin.

There is no need to weigh, measure, count, or plot foods from the lean protein, healthy fat, and neutral vegetable arrows. These foods will not stimulate the insulin roller-coaster. You can eat them whenever you wish.

THE
Arrow Sheet

PROTEIN ARROW
YES
For all steps

(Lean, lite, or low-fat preferred)

cheese
cottage cheese
edamame
egg substitutes
eggs
fish and shellfish
meat
natural seed butter

natural, unsweetened nut butter
poultry
select protein shakes
(1 gram or less net carb grams)
tofu
unsweetened soy milk
white soybeans
or black soybeans

Note: Although meats and cheeses are primarily protein, they vary tremendously in their fat content. The recommended protein sources for the Metabolism Miracle program should be heart healthy and lean. Feel free to enjoy them liberally.

NEUTRAL VEGGIES ARROW
YES
For all steps

artichokes and artichoke hearts
asparagus
bamboo shoots
bean sprouts
beets (½ cup is neutral)
bok choy (pak choy)
broccoli
Brussels sprouts
cabbage
carrots (½ cup sliced, chopped carrots are neutral)
cauliflower

celery
choy sum
cucumbers
delicata squash (1 cup is neutral)
dill pickles
eggplant
green or wax beans
greens (collards, kale, mustard, turnip, spinach)
jicama (1 cup or less is neutral)
kabocha squash (1 cup serving is neutral)

kohlrabi
leeks
lettuce and other salad greens
mushrooms
okra
onions and scallions
peppers (all varieties)
pumpkin (¼ cup is neutral)
radishes
rhubarb
sauerkraut
snap peas

snow peas
spaghetti squash
summer squash
tomatoes (maximum 1 fresh tomato, 10 cherry tomatoes, ½ cup canned tomatoes, ¼ cup sun-dried tomatoes, ½ cup tomato salsa, 4 ounces tomato/vegetable juice is neutral)
turnips
water chestnuts
zucchini

FAT ARROW
YES
For all steps

(Lite or low-fat preferred)

avocado
butter
cream
half-and-half
margarine (butter preferred)
mayonnaise
nuts
oil
olives

salad dressing (with 3 or fewer grams of sugar/2 tablespoons per serving)
seeds (chia, pumpkin, poppy seeds, sesame seeds, sunflower seeds)
sour cream
unsweetened or unsweetened and flavored almond, soy, or coconut milk (or combination)
whipped cream

acorn squash
bread (rolls, buns, bread products)
cereal (hot or cold)
crackers
fruit
fruit juice

granola bars
ice cream and frozen treats
milk
other grains, like wheat, rice, barley, oats
parsnips
pasta

potato chips
potatoes
pretzels
quinoa
regular soda, flavored drinks sweetened with sugar, honey, agave, syrup

rice
sweet potatoes
sweetened beverages
sweets and desserts
winter squash
wraps
yogurt

Dense Carbohydrate Arrow

Full servings are a NO for Step One, but a measured 5-gram net carb portion can be used as a 5-gram Counter Carb in Step One.

Yes for all steps*
5-gram Counter Carbs

Step One: 5-gram Counter Carbs are optional at meals and your bedtime snack. Using 5-gram Counter Carbs appropriately will not slow your weight or inch loss. Eliminating 5-gram Counter Carbs will not increase weight or inch loss.

Steps Two and Three: Count the carb grams as part of your 11- to 20-gram Carb Dam.

*5-gram Counter Carbs must pass the net-carb test and fit the 5-gram Counter Carb rule (page 64). You have the option of using a 5-gram Counter Carb at meals and bedtime.

Net carb grams less than or equal to 1 gram are considered neutral in the serving size of that food.
Net carb grams between 2 and 6 grams are considered a 5-gram Counter Carb.
Remember, sugar-free, no added sugar, reduced sugar, and low-carb verbiage cannot be trusted until you personally check the item's Nutrition Facts.

low-carb beverages
low-carb bread
low-carb candies and treats
low-carb crackers
low-carb milk
low-carb protein drinks with 2 to 6 grams net carb
low-carb tortillas
low-carb wraps
low-carb yogurts

*Foods or recipes in the serving size that provide 6 or fewer grams net carb.

⅓ of an apple, peach, pear, or orange (medium-sized fruit)
⅓ cup blackberries, raspberries, or blueberries

5 cherries
1 puffed Coco Pop™ cake
EAS™ Carb Advantage Shake
14 Goldfish™ crackers
5 grapes
¼ cup mandarin oranges
⅓ cup melon cubes
⅓ cup milk
1 slice Pepperidge Farm™ Carb Style bread
¼ cup pineapple cubes
1 cup popcorn
5 strawberries
2 Triscuit™ crackers
1 Tumaro's™ gourmet low-carb tortilla
5 Wheat Thins™ crackers
⅓ cup plain yogurt

You'll notice a horizontal arrow labeled "5-gram Counter Carbs." A Counter Carb applies to a 5-gram net carb portion of carbohydrate food. They are not the incidental carb grams found in neutral foods like the carb grams in nuts, neutral vegetables, natural peanut butter, or ricotta cheese; 5-gram Counter Carbs contain 5 grams of net carb from foods not normally allowed on Step One, like the 5 grams of net carbohydrate from a certain quantity of fruit, crackers, popcorn, or low-carb products.

On Step One you have the *option* of having a 5-gram Counter Carb at breakfast, lunch, dinner, and bedtime, but the quantity must be limited to 5 grams net carb at each meal and bedtime snack. If you are spacing the 5-gram Counter Carbs out by the clock, keep them four to five hours apart. If 5 grams net carb is eaten too close to the next 5 grams net carb, the total carb grams piggy-back or stack into 10 grams net carb, which *will* cause blood glucose to rise and insulin to release.

So 5 grams net carb at 8:00 a.m. and another 5 grams at 9:00 a.m. counts as 10 grams net carb. These carb grams remain elevated for hours after consumption. This counts as a slip-up on Step One. Consuming 10 grams net carb at once on Step One will reactivate the resting pancreas and liver and set the program back for three entire days.

For ease I suggest you put a 5-gram Counter Carb at your breakfast, lunch, dinner, and bedtime. You needn't use 5-gram Counter Carbs if you don't want to have them; they are optional. If you choose to eliminate these 5-gram Counter Carbs from your program, it will *not* speed weight loss. When it comes to your Counter Carbs, if you don't use them, you lose them. This means that if you don't take your optional 5-gram Counter Carb at breakfast, it's gone. Your next opportunity is at lunch. However, it's okay to have a 5-gram Counter Carb at dinner and another at your bedtime snack *if your bedtime snack is at least two hours after your dinner 5-gram Counter Carb.*

If you prefer to use your 5-gram Counter Carbs by the clock, make sure to time them four to five hours apart.

Although full servings of carbohydrate-dense foods are avoided during Step One, a certain portion of these foods can take the place of a 5-gram Counter Carb; for example, a full serving of fruit (about 15 grams of carb) isn't allowed on Step One, but a 5-gram portion could be used as your 5-gram Counter Carb at meals or bedtime. Remember, a 5-gram Counter Carb can be the 5-gram net carb size of *any* food if the portion equals 2 to 5 grams net carb. Also, the food industry has come up with low-carb versions of many dense-carb foods that fit as Counter Carbs. See page 61 for samples of 5-gram Counter Carbs.

Carb Control

The key to Step One is carbohydrate control. You won't eliminate all carbohydrate foods from your diet, but you'll temporarily avoid or limit most of them. The foods in the protein, fat, and veggie arrows do not require a Nutrition Facts check, even though they contain a limited number of carb grams.

Any carbohydrate above the 5-gram ceiling—half a banana, one slice of whole-grain bread, one container of flavored light yogurt, or an eight-ounce portion of Gatorade—contains about 15 grams of net carb and will alert the pancreas to release insulin, derailing your Step One and landing you right back into metabolic chaos. Keep carb intake under the 5-gram bar at meals and bedtime, and your pancreas will remain in its curative resting state.

So how do you know which foods have 5 or fewer grams of carbohydrates? The carbohydrate grams of the dense carbohydrates to avoid during Step One all exceed the 5-gram limit. But a number of carbohydrate foods can be eaten during Step One. I call these foods 5-gram Counter Carbs because you can tally their carbohydrate total with a quick, easy formula to decide whether they fit the 5-gram rule.

You must be the judge. Never rely on marketing ploys used on the package messaging to tell you the number of carb grams the product contains. You must do the easy math because many food manufacturers make false carbohydrate claims.

You Can Do It

Almost everyone with Metabolism B who sees the "Dense Carbs to Avoid" arrow for Step One goes into a panic. They become pale, shake their heads, and declare, "There is no way I can do this for eight or more weeks!"

This strong reaction to the thought of temporarily avoiding dense-carb foods is just one more affirmation you have uncontrolled Met B. You feel dependent on carb-dense foods. A few notes of encouragement: remember that you *can* have a 5-gram Counter Carb at meals and bedtime, And after day five of Step One your carbohydrate cravings will vanish and you will easily complete the remaining weeks of Step One.

The eight or more weeks of Step One will be a breeze if you follow the 5-gram Counter Carb rule and avoid foods containing more than 6 grams of carbohydrate at meals and bedtime snack. In Step One you have an option to include a 5-gram net Counter Carb at each of your meals, at bedtime, and even in the middle of the night. You can do this without interrupting the new peace your body has found.

Net Carb Grams:
The Simple Formula You Will Use Every Day

It may sound like work to figure out how many carbohydrate grams any particular food has, but it's very straightforward.

An easy formula, the MM net carb formula, is the only one you will need to use during all three steps of the Metabolism Miracle. And you will only use the formula on dense-carb foods or 5-gram Counter Carbs.

The Metabolism Miracle Net Carb Formula
Total carbohydrate grams – dietary fiber grams = net carb grams

To use the formula, look at the Nutrition Facts label on any packaged food. The only numbers you will pay attention to during Step One are:

Serving size
Total carbohydrate grams
Dietary fiber grams

The words "Total Carbohydrate" will always be in dark, bold type on the label. Beneath total carb grams, in lighter type and slightly indented, you will find "Dietary Fiber," along with a slew of other terms, including sugar, other carbs, soluble fiber, insoluble fiber, and sugar alcohol.

In the United States all of the subcategories under the term Total Carbohydrate are already included in the total carb grams. Dietary fiber, although included in the total carb grams, will not convert into blood glucose or tax your pancreas. Dietary fiber cleans the GI tract, lowers cholesterol, and passes, unabsorbed, through your digestive system. A meal or snack with fiber will help you feel full (it adds bulk to your meal), helps slow a rise in blood glucose, can help keep your bowel movements regular, can decrease cholesterol and the risk of GI cancers, and keeps you satisfied between meals. The MM recommendation is finding carb choices (in the starch area) with 2 or more grams of fiber per serving.

Fiber is a carbohydrate, but it is an indigestible carbohydrate. On a food label total carb grams contain the fiber grams, but fiber never converts to blood glucose and never impacts insulin release. Because it isn't part of your Met B issue with carb grams, you need to subtract it out of the total grams. Subtracting the dietary fiber grams from total carbohydrate grams allows you to count only the carb grams that will impact your blood glucose and insulin release. Total carb grams minus dietary fiber grams equal net carb grams. The Metabolism Miracle works with net carb grams.

How to Calculate Net Carbs

Here is an example of how to read a food label and calculate the product's net carbs.

KRAZY KRUNCHY KRISPIES (cereal)

Serving Size 1 cup

Total Carbohydrate 47 grams

   Dietary Fiber 8 grams

Don't pay attention to fat grams, protein grams, sugar grams, or anything else when determining this cereal's net carb grams. You need only subtract away the dietary fiber. Sugar grams are part of the total carb grams.

Subtract the dietary fiber (8 grams) from the total carbohydrate (47 grams), and you have the net carbs (39 grams) for a one-cup serving of this cereal:

$$47 - 8 = 39$$
$$\swarrow \quad \downarrow \quad \searrow$$

total carb – dietary fiber = net carbs

Obviously, with 39 net carb grams per cup, this cereal will *not* fit into Step One of the Metabolism Miracle.

Now, let's look at another example:

AIR-POPPED CORN CRITTERS (cereal)

Serving Size 1 cup

Total Carbohydrate 20 grams

Dietary Fiber 5 grams

$$20 - 5 = 15 \text{ grams net carb in one cup}$$
$$\swarrow \quad \downarrow \quad \searrow$$

total carb – dietary fiber = net carbs

With 15 grams net carb in one cup, one-third cup of this cereal fits into Step One as a 5-gram Counter Carb. Add unsweetened almond or soy milk (neutral), and you can have a nice 5-gram Counter Carb bedtime snack.

Packaged 5-Gram Counter Carbs

Many people miss having bread, crackers, and other traditionally dense carbohydrate foods during Step One of the program. You might consider eating specially designed low-carb versions of these foods, such as low-carb bread, wraps, or tortillas. But don't trust the carb count on the front of the package; instead, always use the MM net carb formula to determine the net carbohydrate grams in a serving, and remember the 5-gram Counter Carb rule. If your low-carb bread contains 7 or more grams of net carb, remove some of the crust to bring it into the 5-gram

BUYER BEWARE

Those tempting whole-grain crackers with their low-carb label may look like they fit into the 5-gram Counter Carb rule, but watch out: marketing on the front of packages can be deceptive. Food companies have different definitions of "low carb" and "sugar-free," and what fits into one low-carb diet may not fit into the Metabolism Miracle's Step One.

The only way to determine whether the crackers have 5 or fewer grams carbohydrate and can fit into Step One is to run a serving size through the net carb formula: total carb grams − dietary fiber grams = net carb. If the net carb is less than 1 gram, it's neutral on MM. If the net carb is 2 to 6 grams, it is a 5-gram Carb Dam.

Serving Size: 6 crackers
Total Carbohydrate: 11 grams
Dietary Fiber: 3 grams
11 − 3 = 8 grams

Keep trying—you'll find another product you love that will have 5 or fewer grams net carb and keep you on the healthy path you've been following. If you insist on having these crackers, four crackers will keep you in the 5-gram Counter Carb zone.

Counter Carb range. You can apply the net carb formula to any foods you're unsure about and, if necessary, reduce your serving size accordingly. The key is to be aware of how many dense carbohydrate grams are on your plate.

Most foods in the protein and healthy fat arrow do not require a 5-gram Counter Carb check. Cheese, cottage cheese, unsweetened natural nut and seed butter, nuts, seeds, olives, avocados, and edamame are in the protein or fat arrows; you need not check their food labels for carb content, as they are considered neutral foods.

Bogus 5-Gram Counter Carbs
There is a list of *bogus* brand-name 5-gram Counter Carbs on www. Miracle-Ville.com. This list cannot be part of this book, as Nutrition Facts change and these products' bogus labeling may change. When you

do the math, you can't make a mistake—but what if the Nutrition Facts or ingredients don't match?

The bogus low-carb foods' Nutrition Facts labeling may fit the 5-gram rule, but their ingredient list might not support their Nutrition Facts. They may cause high blood glucose in those with diabetes and foiled fat burning for those following MM. Check this Bogus list for *your* bread, wrap, yogurt, pasta, and so forth, and if you find it on the list, stop using it. (The website also has a list of brand-name products that truly are 5-gram Counter Carbs.)

If you have been using a bogus product, you should stop using it, but finish your eight weeks on Step One.

Reweigh and remeasure on schedule. If you haven't reached your expected pounds/inches at the end of the eighth week, continue with Step One using an honest product. Once you reach your expected fat and inches, you will move on to Step Two.

What About Sugar Alcohol?

When reading an ingredient list of products labeled "sugar-free," "low sugar," or "low carb," you'll often come across ingredients that end in the letters "-ol" such as mannitol, xylitol, and sorbitol. Ingredients ending in -ol are most likely sugar alcohols. These ingredients are *not* calorie-free. They have less impact on blood glucose than actual sugar because they are not completely absorbed in the GI tract. Because they don't fully absorb, sugar alcohol ferments in the large intestine and can cause bloating, gas, flatulence, and diarrhea. *Don't ever* subtract sugar or most sugar alcohol grams from total carb grams of carbohydrate—unless it is erythritol.

Erythritol is the only sugar alcohol that must be subtracted from total carb grams.

Erythritol is a sugar alcohol that works differently from all the others. It's considered to be noncaloric and has no impact on blood glucose or insulin release. (For more about erythritol, see Sugar Substitutes, page 70).

So if a Nutrition Facts Label contains the sugar alcohol erythritol, subtract the erythritol!

Serving Size ½ cup
Total Carbohydrate 18 grams
Dietary Fiber 4 grams
Sugar Alcohol (erythritol) 6 grams
Sugar 8 grams

The net carb grams would be: total carb grams – dietary fiber grams – erythritol grams = net carb grams.

$$18 - 4 - 6 = 8 \text{ grams net carb}$$

On the following nutrition label a sugar alcohol other than erythritol is used. If mannitol, xylitol, sorbitol, or isomalt appears in the ingredient list, do not subtract the sugar alcohol grams.

Serving Size ½ cup	
Total Carbohydrate 18 grams	
Dietary Fiber 4 grams	
Sugar Alcohol (sorbitol) 6 grams	
Sugar 8 grams	

The net carb grams would be: total carb grams − dietary fiber = net carb grams

$$18 - 4 = 14 \text{ grams net carb}$$

If you see sugar alcohol grams on Nutrition Facts without the name of the sugar alcohol listed, check the package's ingredient list to find the sugar alcohol that's been used. (Chances are the sugar alcohol will end in -ol.)

Sugar Substitutes

Erythritol (Swerve)

Erythritol occurs naturally in grapes, melons, and pears. Since 1990 erythritol has been made through natural fermentation and can be added to foods and beverages to provide sweetness and bulk without adding calories. Some brand names for erythritol are Swerve™, ZSweet™, and Zerose™. Erythritol can also be purchased in health food stores and comes in granulated or powdered forms.

Erythritol is a natural sweetener that measures cup-for-cup like sugar in recipes. It has no bitter aftertaste, zero calories, causes no rise in blood glucose, and is non-GMO. Erythritol has the ability to brown and caramelize.

Its total carb content is 5 grams per teaspoon, but these grams get subtracted from total carb grams because it prompts no rise in blood glucose or insulin. Erythritol has no risk of GI side effects such as gas, abdominal distention, diarrhea, or flatulence that can occur with other sugar alcohols like sorbitol, xylitol, mannitol, or isomalt.

Erythritol sugar replacements have a combination of erythritol and oligosaccharides that provide excellent baking and cooking functionality. Oligosaccharides are nondigestible carbs that act like fiber or a

READING AN EU LABEL

The MM Nutrition Facts label reading tutorial is based on reading a US packaged food or food product. If you are reading a food label with European Union (EU) labeling, please take note.

The following categories are now mandatory on EU food labels:

1. Calories: energy value (in both kilojoules [kJ] and kilocalories [kcal])
2. Grams of fat
3. Grams of saturated fat
4. Grams of carbohydrate
5. Grams of sugar
6. Grams of protein
7. Grams of salt

The following are considered *voluntary* components of EU food labeling. They need not appear on packaged foods and are optional in food labeling.

1. Grams of monounsaturates
2. Grams of polyunsaturates
3. Grams of polyols (sugar alcohol grams)
4. Grams of starch
5. Grams of fibre
6. Certain vitamins and minerals

If you are reading EU food labels, be certain to check the serving size and then move on to grams of carbohydrate. The food label will not necessarily list grams of fiber. *On an EU label fiber grams have already been subtracted from Carbohydrate grams; the Total Carbohydrate grams are the net carb grams.*

On the negative side, fiber and polyol (sugar alcohol) grams are not mandatory. You won't always know if fiber grams are 2 or more grams or if sugar alcohols have been used in the product. If mannitol, xylitol, sorbitol, or isomalt are in the ingredients, don't subtract them from carbohydrate grams. If erythritol is the sugar alcohol in the item, its grams need to be subtracted.

In short, EU labels focus on carbohydrate grams—these grams are actually shown as net carb grams with dietary fiber already subtracted. If polyols (sugar alcohols) are listed in Nutrition Facts, look to the ingredient list to check for the *type* of polyol. If erythritol is the sugar alcohol (polyol) in the product, subtract polyol grams from carbohydrate grams.

prebiotic in the large intestine. Erythritol sugar replacements actually help keep the gut healthy!

Stevia

Stevia is also a replacement for sugar. Some think stevia has a unique bitter aftertaste similar to licorice. I find it a good nonsugar sweetener for beverages like coffee, tea, iced tea, or iced coffee or to sweeten foods with a more fluid consistency like plain yogurt, hot cereal, or pudding.

and a dab of mayonnaise. She poured a glass of green tea with stevia and lemon and sat down to eat. When she was through she felt satisfied. After an outdoor walk with coworkers she returned to work for the afternoon.

As the afternoon wore on, Brenda started to feel tired and a little cranky. She yearned for that mini chocolate bar and a cup of coffee. She caught herself and realized, This is happening because my liver is releasing glycogen stores and my brain is coaxing me to eat carbohydrates to hike up my blood glucose. She grabbed another handful of those chocolate-flavored almonds and a cup of coffee.

After work Brenda got home and suddenly felt famished. It was five hours since lunch. She chose to have a 5-gram Counter Carb in the form of a low-carb protein shake. And after relaxing and drinking the shake, she felt satisfied and ready to put together a quick dinner. She put a salmon steak on her counter-top grill, steamed some broccoli, and dropped a dab of whipped butter on her "faux" mashed potatoes (page 318).

At around 9:00 p.m. Brenda was yearning for something sweet. She grabbed two containers of sugar-free gelatin, topped each with whipped cream, and enjoyed every sweet bite.

Right before bed she had her last 5-gram Counter Carb: a slice of low-carb whole-grain toast with natural almond butter and carb-free jelly. After her nightly cup of chamomile tea, Brenda was off to bed, feeling positive about Step One. *I can do this,* she thought right before she fell asleep.

In a blink day five of Step One arrived. Sure enough, Brenda woke up with great energy and looked less puffy and bloated. A big smile came to her face: *I CAN do this.*

Stevia contains zero calories, zero glycemic index, and no carb grams. Like erythritol, it has no impact on blood glucose levels or insulin release. It's extremely sweet and a little goes a long way. There are different types of stevia; some are pure stevia powder with no bulking agent, others come in liquid form, and others have additions of bulking agents like maltodextrin or inulin (not to be confused with insulin) that do not impact blood glucose or insulin release. These bulking agents make measuring the amount of stevia to use almost the same as sugar.

Stevia used for baking can lead to many trial-and-error attempts to "get it right." You need to use a conversion chart when replacing sugar with stevia in a recipe. Your brand of stevia should have a conversion table for the product that clearly shows how much of the stevia product to use in place of sugar.

For the sake of understanding the conversion of one commonly found brand of stevia, Sweetleaf™, I have included some recipes that incorporate Sweetleaf and Sweetleaf's conversion chart. Again, remember to check the conversion chart on the particular brand of stevia you choose.

Stevia and Erythritol Blend (Truvia)

Truvia™ is a blend of erythritol and stevia, with natural flavor. Packet for packet, Truvia measures the same as Splenda, but when you use spoonable Truvia the conversion gets trickier (three-quarters of a teaspoon of the spoonable product contains the same level of sweetness as a packet of Truvia).

Sucralose (Splenda)

Splenda™ is the only non-nutritive sweetener that starts out as table sugar, or sucrose. During processing three oxygen-hydrogen groups on the sugar molecule are replaced with three chlorine atoms to create a totally new molecule. Due to replacing oxygen-hydrogen groups with chlorine atoms, sucralose is considered an artificial sweetener. Splenda was developed in 1976. It is now approved in more than eighty countries and is used worldwide in thousands of commercial products such as no-sugar-added fruit, diet soft drinks, and reduced-sugar juices, jelly, and ice cream.

More than one hundred studies over twenty years have demonstrated that sucralose is not responsible for negative health effects such as cancer or birth defects. Unlike sugar, Splenda is not fully metabolized; the majority leaves the body in the feces and a small amount exits through the urine.

Splenda is considered safe for everyone, including pregnant and nursing women and children. People with diabetes can use it safely because it does not affect carbohydrate metabolism or insulin levels. Because the body cannot digest or absorb all the sucralose, it provides no appreciable calories. The FDA's accepted daily intake level is 5 mg/kg of body weight. This is roughly the equivalent of 25 packets of Splenda per day or six cans of diet soft drinks.

Splenda does not promote tooth decay. It is so sweet—about six hundred times sweeter than sugar—that a bulking agent like maltodextrin is added to sucralose to make its measurement close to that of sugar in recipes. Although Splenda provides a sweet taste similar to that of sugar, it does not contribute to baked goods' browning. As a result, products baked with Splenda may not brown during baking and will stale faster.

There are so many sugar substitutes on the market. The following decisions regarding MM friendliness are based on my research. Use it as a guide when you choose your sugar substitute.

Artificial Sweeteners: MM friendly?
    acesulfame potassium or acesulfame K: yes
    aspartame (Equal, Nutrasweet): no
    neotame: no
    saccharin (Sweet'N Low™, Sugar Twin™): no
    sucralose (Splenda): yes

Sugar Alcohols: MM friendly?
    (sugar alcohol grams are part of the total carb grams)
    erythritol (preferred): yes
    isomalt: yes
    lactilol: yes
    malitol: yes
    mannitol: yes
    sorbitol: yes
    xylitol: yes

Novel sweeteners: MM friendly?
    stevia: yes
    neotame: no (contains aspartame)
    tagatose (Tagatesse™, European): yes
    advantame: no (contains aspartame)

Now that you have a sense of the easy carb counting you'll do on Step One, take enjoyment from the fact that you won't have to count a thing in the lean proteins, healthy fat, and neutral vegetable categories. There is no food weighing, measuring, or counting of neutral foods on the Metabolism Miracle program. Have them anytime in reasonable quantities, and you'll continue to lose weight and feel great.

The Protein-Fat Pack:
Meat, Cheese, Nuts, and More

Consider higher-fat meat and protein to have a yellow light: proceed with caution.

As Steps One and Two are designed to set your body into fat-burning mode, it's important not to add excess fat to your daily dietary intake. An occasional higher-fat meat choice is acceptable, but most of your protein choices should be of the lean or low-fat variety.

Lean proteins have the green light on MM, so eat them liberally. Skinless poultry, lean cuts of beef, reduced-fat cheese, egg whites, soy products, and other proteins will provide your body with high biological value protein and a sense of satisfaction and fullness. Prime rib and sirloin are both proteins, and the sirloin's low-fat profile gives it a place on the recommended protein list. Your body will always burn the fat from the foods you eat before it will burn your fat stores. The sirloin will help you take full advantage of your body's new fat-burning mode.

When you choose lean proteins, healthy fats, and neutral vegetables found on the arrow list, you won't have to concern yourself with serving sizes. You can, on occasion, choose a protein with a higher fat content. Just remember that after day five of your program your body has transitioned to fat-burning mode, and you should take full advantage by choosing lean or light proteins; your body won't waste time burning fat from food and will focus on burning your excess fat stores. This will make the difference in your inches and the size of your clothing.

The same holds true for added fats. You can use light or regular fats (*no* fat-free versions), but the same amount of regular salad dressing and

BE CAREFUL WITH LOW-CARB RECIPES

As you peruse cookbooks or the Internet for low-carb choices, you will quickly notice that most low-carb recipes exceed the Step One limit for the Metabolism Miracle. Even recipes designed for other low-carb programs will rarely fit MM's Step One. The issue is that all other low-carb diets count *every single carb gram,* even in foods the Metabolism Miracle program considers neutral. As a result, a recipe containing shrimp, neutral veggies, garlic, butter, and white wine would list all the carb grams in all the ingredients. On MM the entire dish would be neutral!

When in doubt, stay with the recipes in *The Metabolism Miracle; The Metabolism Miracle Cookbook; The Metabolism Miracle, Second Edition,* or any of the new and converted recipes on www.Miracle-Ville.com.

light salad dressing may contain very different amounts of fat. They are both neutral, but using less regular dressing or a regular amount of light salad dressing is the way to go.

Many newbies to the Metabolism Miracle are afraid to begin the program. Although they are hopeful that this program will work for them, they fear not being able to "do it" or that they will make a mistake and blow their last chance at weight loss and better health. Before beginning, you might peek in your kitchen cabinets and see carb foods everywhere: cereal, crackers, chips, pretzels, pasta, rice, baked beans, cookies, sugar, honey, and more. If you live alone, consider bagging packaged carb-dense foods for the duration of Step One. If you live with others who are not on the program, put all the off-limits dense-carb items in their own cabinet so others can have easy access but you can ignore them.

Flour Substitutes

Breads and baked goods are among the foods people on Step One miss the most. Most baked goods and breads contain the dense carbohydrate wheat flour. The following flour substitutes can be used in baking and are *neutral* on MM.

Almond Flour

Blanched almond flour is very finely ground and will *not* contain the skins from the almonds. Substitute 1:1 for wheat flour in recipes.

Soy Flour

Soy flour is best suited for use in combination with another neutral flour in a baked recipe, as by itself it may have a strong taste. Stir soy flour before using. Measure out three-quarters of a cup of soy flour for every one cup of flour called for in the recipe. For two cups of regular flour, use three-quarters cup of soy flour and one and one-quarter cups of almond flour.

Coconut Flour

Using coconut flour is *not* a simple 1:1 replacement for regular flour in baking. You may have best results using recipes that already call for coconut flour instead of trying to substitute! Coconut flour is very high in fiber and absorbs large amounts of liquid. Batters made with coconut flour will not resemble those made with wheat flour. Let the batter sit for a few minutes and remember that the liquid will be absorbed further in the baking process. Always sift coconut flour before using.

Coconut flour can replace up to 20 percent of the total flour in a recipe, and remember to add 20 percent more liquid to the recipe for the added coconut flour.

For every cup of wheat flour in a recipe, use one-quarter cup coconut flour, three-quarter cup almond or soy flour, double the eggs, and add an extra one-third cup of liquid, such as water or unsweetened almond milk.

Flax Meal or Flaxseed Flour

You can replace 25 percent of the flour in a baked good recipe with flaxseed flour. Choose either soy or almond flour for the other 75 percent.

The "Yes" Lists: Neutral on All Steps of MM

Lean Proteins

Choose mainly lean proteins during *any* step of the Metabolism Miracle.

TAKE OFF YOUR COAT . . . AND CHECK YOUR SAUCE

You may use any cooking method except those that incorporate coating, breading, flour, bread crumbs, sweetened sauces, gravies, or sweet marinades.

Grilling, baking, roasting, sautéing, and broiling all pass muster with the Metabolism Miracle plan. For additional flavor, use herbs, spices, and seasonings. Some reputable low-carb food purveyors make special breading mixes with neutral flours other than wheat flour.

Breading made with almond flour, flax meal, soy flour, or coconut flour can be neutral. Low-carb bread crumbs are available but might need to be used as your 5-gram Counter Carb. Some jarred gravies contain zero grams net carb.

Xanthan Gum

When making your own sauces, soups, and sauces, you may try xanthan gum as a neutral thickener. To use xanthan gum, use about one-eighth teaspoon per cup of liquid, and combine these in a blender or with an immersion blender—not by hand, as it will "gum" almost instantly and form clumps if not constantly in motion while it is incorporated into the liquid.

Another method of adding xanthan gum to your sauces or gravies is to use a fine-mesh tea strainer/infuser. Simply add the desired amount of xanthan gum into the tea infuser and snap the lid tightly closed. Then shake the xanthan powder over the liquid to be thickened, stirring gently with one hand while shaking or "sifting" the infuser. The xanthan gum falls in such a fine powder that it doesn't clump at all. This method also makes it very easy to adjust the amount you need, as you can add more or less as it thickens in the pan. If any is left over in the infuser, you can dump it back into the container.

Beef

Because most people with uncontrolled Metabolism B have elevated LDL cholesterol, their health care provider typically advises them to limit or avoid red meat. However, lean cuts of red meat are fine to enjoy on a regular basis. In any case, always trim any visible fat.

chuck roast	porterhouse steak
filet mignon	round steak
flank steak	rump roast
ground beef (85–93 percent)	sirloin
ground round	T-bone steak
London broil	tenderloin rib roast

Fish and Shellfish

All varieties of fish and shellfish are neutral. Eat fish and seafood broiled, grilled, boiled, or steamed, and omit breading, coating, or cocktail sauce. Avoid artificial seafood; companies add carbohydrate grams to the fish, and it is not a neutral protein choice.

clams	salmon
cod	sardines
crab	scallops
flounder	sea bass
haddock	shrimp
halibut	snapper
herring (not creamed)	swordfish
lobster	tilapia
mahi-mahi	trout
oysters	tuna (fresh or canned in water)
pollock	whiting

Lamb, Veal, and Game

Trim all visible fat.

buffalo	roast lamb
deer	skinless duck (naturally higher
lamb chop	in fat than chicken)
lean veal chop	skinless pheasant
leg of lamb	veal roast
ostrich	venison

Pork

Most cuts of pork are lean, but pork products such as sausage, deli meats, pepperoni, and sausage patties contain added fat.

Canadian bacon
canned, cured, or boiled ham
center-cut loin chops
deli ham

fresh ham
pork tenderloin
trimmed pork chops

Poultry

Be sure to remove skin from poultry. Processed turkey products are higher in fat content, so limit their use: turkey bacon, turkey sausage, turkey pepperoni, turkey burgers, and turkey kielbasa all have a higher fat content than turkey itself, so limit their use.

chicken (white meat, skinless)
Cornish game hen

turkey (white meat, skinless)

Cheese

Cheese that has 5 or fewer grams of fat per ounce is considered lower-fat cheese.

grated cheese, such as
　　Parmesan and Romano
low-fat cheese

low-fat cottage cheese
part-skim ricotta, mozzarella,
　　and string cheese

By nature, cheese is a high-fat food. When possible choose low-fat or light cheese, cream cheese, ricotta, and cottage cheese. (If cheese has 5 or fewer grams of fat per ounce, it is considered a low-fat or light choice.) Low-fat cheeses are preferred over fat-free choices because the latter have more additives, tend to be plastic-like in texture, and do not melt. The serving size of cheese is 1 ounce.

You may eat regular (full-fat) cheese, but be aware that your body will spend time burning the fat from the cheese instead of the fat off your body. Restaurants rarely carry low-fat cheese, so you may choose to have regular cheese when eating out, but stock your home or office refrigerator with the lower-fat variety.

Eggs

Eat as many egg whites or as much egg substitute as you like, as they are great sources of lean protein with no fat. Try to limit your use of whole eggs, as each egg naturally contains the fat grams of one pat or one teaspoon of butter. For example, when making an omelet, use two or three egg whites but only one of the yolks.

egg substitute (fat free)	whole eggs (contain about 5
egg whites (fat free)	grams of fat per egg)

Soy and Soy Products

Meat substitutes sometimes contain added grain, corn, peas, and legumes. Veggie burgers and meat replacement products that contain 5 or fewer grams net carbohydrate are neutral. You may have more than one serving, and they will remain neutral. If your soy-based meat alternative has more than 6 grams net carb per serving, the carb grams must be counted and the meat alternative is not neutral.

edamame	vegetarian or soy-based meat
tofu	substitutes with fewer than
unsweetened soy milk	5 grams net carb per serving

Peanut and Nut Butters

Natural peanut, almond, or cashew butter, containing only nuts and optional salt as ingredients, offers the best choice during Step One because most processed peanut butter is sweetened with sugar. Just as you don't

---

SWEETENED PEANUT BUTTER

If you miss the taste of your sweet and creamy childhood peanut butters, which were often hydrogenated and sugar sweetened, try making your own without trans fats and sugar.

1. Make sure your natural nut butter contains nothing but nuts, oil, and perhaps salt. There must be no added sweetener like honey or sugar in any form.
2. Remove the top from the natural peanut butter jar.
3. Microwave for about thirty seconds to soften the peanut butter.
4. Stir in a packet of sucralose (Splenda), stevia, or erythritol (Swerve) and, if desired, a pinch of salt until totally blended.
5. Store in the refrigerator.

---

have to be concerned about the carb content of nuts, you don't have to count the carb grams in natural, unsweetened peanut butter. Processed peanut butter, like Skippy™ or Peter Pan™, has added sugar and counts as a 5-gram Counter Carb; remember to measure the amount listed as the serving size for 5 grams net carb.

> natural almond or cashew butter with no added sugar (refrigerate after opening)
>
> natural peanut butter with no added sugar (refrigerate after opening)
>
> processed peanut butter or nut butters (use 5-gram Counter Carb rule)

Reduced-Carbohydrate Protein Shakes

These premixed ready-to-drink shakes contain the protein of about 3 ounces of meat per serving along with added vitamins and minerals. You can find them in the supermarket or pharmacy.

> Net carb grams = 1 gram or less per shake is neutral.
>
> If net carb grams are 2 to 6 grams per serving, count as a 5-gram Counter Carb.

Healthier Fats: Avoid Fat-Free Fat

butter

butter blends (half butter, half healthy oil)

light or low-fat butter

light or low-fat cream cheese

light or low-fat mayonnaise

light or low-fat salad dressing with 3 or fewer grams sugar

light or low-fat sour cream

light, tub, and whipped margarines (avoid hydrogenation and trans fat)

whipped butter

For years butter had a bad reputation because it is made from the saturated fat of milk. Margarine, however, is made of vegetable oil, not saturated fat with cholesterol and animal fat. On the surface, oil seems like a healthier alternative to the use of a saturated fat, right? Wrong.

The healthy oil used in margarine was made spreadable by pumping in hydrogen. This process is called hydrogenation. Hydrogenation breaks apart oil's fat chains and releases substances called free radicals, or trans fats. Trans fat intake has been linked to cancer. Note the rise in stomach and colon cancer from the advent of margarine, vegetable shortening, creamy peanut butter, and mass-produced baked goods containing hydrogenated fat after the late 1940s.

If you are choosing margarine or spread, look for a product that contains no trans fats or hydrogenated fat. Also, avoid partial hydrogenation. The first ingredient should be liquid oil, not partially hydrogenated oil.

Oils

- canola oil
- coconut oil
- corn oil
- flaxseed oil
- olive oil
- peanut oil
- safflower oil
- sunflower oil
- vegetable oil

Salad Dressings*

Most unsweetened regular dressings contain a very small amount of carbohydrate, and vinaigrettes contain even less. Use regular salad dressing in a sparing amount; the salad dressing may be neutral, but it is high in fat. The age-old technique of taking salad on your fork and dipping it lightly into your salad dressing on the side really does help cut down on your total fat consumption.

Light or low-fat dressings also work with the Metabolism Miracle.

Avoid fat-free salad dressings. These dressings need to replace the flavor that is lost when the manufacturer removes all the fat. Unfortunately, flavor is replaced by adding more sugar and more carb grams than regular or light dressing.

*The Salad Dressing Rule: When choosing a salad dressing, make certain the dressing's *sugar* grams are 3 or fewer grams per two tablespoons of dressing.

Mayonnaise

Light or low-fat is preferred. If using regular mayonnaise, use less.

Olives

Enjoy green, black, and stuffed olives.

Nuts

Almonds, cashews, pecans, pistachios, and walnuts are all good choices. Peanuts (technically legumes) are also neutral.

Avoid honey-roasted nuts or nuts sprinkled with flavors, as the honey or added sugar makes them count as 5-gram Counter Carbs.

Further, people with a history of diverticulosis, ulcerative colitis, or stomach and GI upset should check with their healthcare provider to see whether nuts are recommended based on their medical condition. Your physician might advise that you chew nuts into a smooth paste before swallowing.

A handful of nuts in the midmorning, midafternoon, and evening can be a great choice of snack. Although they contain carbohydrate, the healthy fat content of nuts slows their digestion, causing the carbohydrate to be released so slowly that it is negligible to your blood glucose. Spread your intake of nuts throughout the day, and don't go overboard with the quantity. (I once had a patient who consumed a five-pound bag of pistachios in one afternoon. She called the office in the late afternoon, complaining of stomach pains!) Three handfuls per day is a good rule of thumb when it comes to your intake of nuts. Consuming an excessive amount of nuts leads to an excessive fat intake and, thus, difficulty burning the fat on your body and in your blood. Some of the MM recipes use nut and seed flours in place of carb-dense wheat flour. If you have one dessert/day and it contains almond flour or flax meal, deduct one handful of nuts for the day.

Seeds
   chia seeds
   poppy seeds
   pumpkin seeds
   sesame seeds
   sunflower seeds
   tahini paste (ground sesame seeds)

Avocado

Avocado has heart-healthy monounsaturated fats, but keep in mind that one avocado has the fat content of eight teaspoons of butter and almost five hundred calories.

NEUTRAL MILK SUBSTITUTES:
UNSWEETENED SOY MILK OR ALMOND MILK

Almond and soy milk are both plant-based dairy substitutes. For a variety of reasons many people choose unsweetened soy or almond milk over dairy (cow's) milk.

Allergies. People who are allergic to milk (may be allergic to lactose, casein, or whey) avoid cow's milk and yogurt due to their allergies. Both unsweetened almond and soy milk can take the place of regular milk in a 1:1 replacement ratio in recipes and can be used as beverages or in cereals.

Cholesterol. Cow's milk contains cholesterol. If you're restricting cholesterol, you might prefer to use soy or almond milk because they are cholesterol-free.

Blood Sugar Impact. Neither unsweetened soy nor almond milk has a significant impact on insulin or blood sugar. Although soy milk is derived from a legume and almond milk from a nut, for our purposes they are considered to be neutral. Cow's milk is a carbohydrate choice.

Hormones and Antibiotics. Cow's milk may contain hormones or antibiotics from the cow's feed source.

Unsweetened Soy Milk

Soy milk has as much protein as dairy milk, is low in fat, and contains no cholesterol. It's a good source of iron and can be fortified with calcium.

However, there are some health conditions that may be adversely affected by the consumption of soy, but keep in mind that the negative health consequences linked to soy consumption are not related to a normal intake of soy; they are based on a very high intake of soy. If vegans are concerned because their main protein source is soy, they can get protein from non-soy sources, including grains, legumes, nuts and nut butters, and enriched cereals.

- Testosterone levels and infertility: Soy contains isoflavones (proteins). A high intake of isoflavone has been linked to decreased sperm concentration and testosterone levels in male monkeys. Ask your MD about your case.
- Breast Cancer: Soy milk contains phytoestrogen, a plant hormone similar to estrogen, and articles have linked soy to breast cancer. Researchers at the Mayo Clinic reviewed all the evidence and concluded that soy has not been shown to fuel breast cancer cells. Phytoestrogens may reduce the effectiveness of tamoxifen (a breast cancer medication), and research from the University of Maryland Medical Center recommends those taking tamoxifen should avoid soy. Ask your MD regarding your case.
- Thyroid issues: Isoflavones may lower iodine levels, which can decrease functioning of the thyroid gland. Soy milk may also interfere with the body's ability to absorb thyroid medication and may cause issues if there is iodine deficiency. (In the US, most people consume iodized salt, which balances out any iodine lost from soy consumption). You may want to use soy in limited amounts if you have thyroid issues. Ask your MD about your case.

Unsweetened Almond Milk

Almond milk is the white liquid made by soaking, blending, and straining almonds. Unlike the distinct flavor of soy milk, almond milk has a mild, nutty flavor that most people enjoy. You might consider avoiding almond milk if you have a peach or tree nut allergy. Ask your MD about your case.

Almond milk comes unsweetened, sweetened, and flavored/unsweetened. Those with Metabolism B should use the unsweetened versions to keep carbohydrate content down. Almond milk has lower protein content than soy or cow's milk, but it is a good source of iron, Vitamin D, and Vitamin E. Most almond milk manufacturers fortify their milk with calcium. Almond milk contains omega 3 fatty acids, which may help decrease cholesterol and blood pressure and protect against cardiovascular and neurological disease.

HOW MUCH IS TOO MUCH?

Tammy tends to take things literally. She was determined to follow MM by the book, and because natural peanut butter is in the protein arrow and is a neutral, she decided she could use it in any quantity. She used about three-fourths of a jar every day for her toast, by the spoonful, and in her protein shake.

After eight weeks on Step One Tammy looked great, felt great, and had significant improvements in her blood pressure and lab work. But when she compared her starting weight and measurements at the end of her eighth week, she had lost less than her expected weight/inch loss of fourteen to twenty-one pounds.

I checked her food log and noticed the excessive use of natural peanut butter, regular cheese, butter, and whole avocados. I explained that although the majority of her excess weight was due to her uncontrolled Met B, extra-large portions of high-fat proteins and regular fats also contribute to her weight. If she consumed an excess quantity of protein and fat, her body would have no choice but to store the excess as fat.

For that reason, unlike some other low-carb diets, the Metabolism Miracle will never suggest that you eat a quarter-pound of bacon, drench your salad in blue cheese dressing, or smother your broccoli with heaping spoonfuls of butter. But you can have Canadian bacon, balsamic vinaigrette, and broccoli with a touch of whipped butter and continue to lose fat and weight.

Use common sense and consume normal portions of lean protein, heart-healthy fat, and low-carb veggies.

Sour Cream or Cream Cheese
Light or reduced fat is recommended. Use less if you are using the whole-fat variety.

Creamer or Half-and-Half
Light or low-fat is recommended. Use regular cream or half-and-half sparingly due to fat content. When using flavored creamers, check against the net carb test and count them as a 5-gram Counter Carb.

Neutral Vegetables

Go to town eating the following vegetables. With the exception of beets, carrots, tomatoes, and tomato products that must be limited (see Tomato Tip, page 90), you may eat the other neutral vegetables at any time and in any quantity, even during Step One. They are filled with vitamins, minerals, fiber, and antioxidants for great health but have minimal impact on blood glucose or insulin release.

artichokes and artichoke hearts
asparagus
bamboo shoots
bean sprouts
beets (½ cup is neutral)
bok choy (pak choy)
broccoli
Brussels sprouts
cabbage
carrots (½ cup chopped or
    sliced carrots are neutral)
cauliflower
celery
choy sum
cucumbers
delicata squash (1 cup or less
    is neutral)
dill pickles
eggplant
green or wax beans
greens (collards, kale, mustard,
    turnip, spinach)
jicama (1 cup or less is neutral)
kabocha squash (1 cup or less is
    neutral)
kohlrabi
leeks

lettuce and other salad greens
mushrooms
okra
onions and scallions
peppers (all varieties)
pumpkin (¼ cup is neutral)
radishes
rhubarb
sauerkraut
snap peas
snow peas
spaghetti squash
summer squash
tomatoes (maximum 1 fresh
    tomato, 10 cherry tomatoes,
    ½ cup of canned tomatoes,
    ¼ cup of sun dried tomatoes,
    ½ cup of tomato salsa,
    4 ounces of tomato/
    vegetable juice is neutral)
turnips
water chestnuts
zucchini

Think of tomatoes as a cross between a fruit and a vegetable. They contain more carb grams than other neutral vegetables. See the vegetable list for the maximum allowable portions to be considered neutral on Step One.

Most commercial or prepared tomato sauce is not allowed during Step One, as it contains added sugar or concentrated tomato paste. Consider making a quick marinara sauce of crushed tomatoes, minced garlic, finely chopped onion, wine, and olive oil. A half-cup serving of this sauce is permitted on Step One as a 5-gram Counter Carb.

If you find a brand of marinara sauce that contains tomatoes, herbs, and spices only, a half cup is neutral.

Other Neutral Foods

During Step One you can have these foods whenever you like as long as their net carb grams are 1 gram or less.

Neutral Sweets

Maximum one serving of dessert per day. Remember, your body will burn the fat from what you eat before it burns the fat from your body. Don't let excess neutral desserts slow up your progress.

carb-free jelly (most sugar-free jelly fits into the 5-gram Counter Carb territory)

carb-free syrup (most sugar-free syrup fits into the 5-gram Counter Carb territory)

sugar-free chewing gum

sugar-free gelatin (most contain aspartame, so use in moderation)

Basics

bouillon consommé

broth

Neutral Beverages

club soda coffee

*diet or sugar-free soda
*select fitness water, flavored
    waters, and flavored seltzers

sugar-free tonic
tea

*For diet soda or flavored beverages, choose those without aspartame. Choose one with sucralose, stevia, or erythritol as the sweetener.

Condiments
dill pickles
herbs
lemon and lime juice
mustard

spices
vinegar
white horseradish

What About Alcoholic Beverages?

Most alcoholic beverages begin with fruit or grain. Before it is fermented or distilled, the fruit or grain is a dense carbohydrate. For this reason people assume wine and spirits are mainly carbohydrate. But once fermented or distilled, the dense carbs undergo a chemical change into alcohol that the body does not treat as a carb-dense food. Unsweetened alcohol does not cause a spike in blood glucose and is, in fact, treated like fat in the body. (Regular beer is not the same—see below for more detail.)

One drink is defined as:

1.5 ounces of spirits = 2 teaspoons fat (about 100 fat calories)
12 ounces of light beer = 2 teaspoons fat (about 100 fat calories)
5 ounces of unsweetened wine = 2 teaspoons fat (about 100 fat calories)

Keep in mind that after day five of Step One your liver is on a temporary vacation and may be slower to process alcohol.

The liver has an important function when it comes to alcoholic beverages, as it is responsible for clearing alcohol (as well as most medications and toxins) from the bloodstream. During Step One, while the liver rests, its blood-cleaning mechanism may run slower than normal. Perhaps this is why those who are following Step One feel alcohol's effects faster and for a longer time than when their Met B was out of control. So

FUDGING NUTRITION FACTS

One brand of ice pop features the Splenda logo. The label states, "Use for low-carb diets," and on the front it states, "4 grams of net carb!" The pops seem perfect for Step One, right? Look again, this time with the net carb formula to help you:

Serving Size 1 ice pop

Total Carbohydrate 12 grams

Dietary Fiber 4 grams

Sugar 4 grams

Sugar Alcohol 4 grams

The sugar alcohol is *not* erythritol, so it *cannot* be subtracted from total carb grams.

12 grams (total carb) – 4 grams (dietary fiber) = 8 grams (net carbs)

Companies get away with faulty math because the FDA currently has no set formula for net carb. The ice pop manufacturer subtracted *both* the dietary fiber *and* the sugar alcohol grams to come up with the 4 grams net carb listed on the front of the package. But sugar alcohol, with the exception of erythritol, cannot be subtracted from total carb grams. If you trusted the marketing statement on the front of the package, your pancreas would release insulin and set you back for three days.

Many low-carb products on your store's shelves similarly misrepresent the net carb grams on the front of their packages. Always use the net carb formula to protect yourself.

although one or two drinks in a night will probably fit into Step One of the Metabolism Miracle, please drink alcohol wisely and slowly to feel its effect before continuing. And check with your MD regarding drinking alcohol with your medical history and medications.

Be sure to consult your physician regarding alcohol because certain medications and health conditions such as diabetes can change your reaction to alcohol. Medications for metabolic syndrome may also interact with alcohol. Every person's situation is different. On the Metabolism

Miracle program the *maximum* amount of alcohol—and only with physician approval—is one or two alcohol-containing beverages per day.

Distilled Spirits (vodka, rum, whiskey, gin, etc.) are neutral in and of themselves. However, mixers are often sugary, so watch their carb content.

Carb-free Mixers: For mixing or chasing, you have the following neutral options:

- carb-free water flavor mixers like Propel™ powder (no aspartame)
- diet sodas (no aspartame)
- diet tonic water (no aspartame)
- seltzer water
- soda water
- sparkling water (like Perrier™)

Liqueur: Avoid liqueurs such as Amaretto™, Bailey's™, crème de cacao, Grand Marnier™, ouzo, sambuca, Kahlua™, triple sec, Cointreau™, kirsch, Campari™, or crème de menthe, as they almost always contain added sugar and carb grams.

Beer: In order to be neutral, a beer must be a light beer. No regular beer, red or dark ale, or stout. Drink no more than two twelve-ounce servings of light beer per day.

Neutral Wine
- Cabernet Sauvignon
- Champagne/sparkling wine
- Chardonnay
- merlot

pinot grigio   Sauvignon blanc
pinot noir

Avoid sweetened wines like sangria, as sweetened wines are wine plus
sugar.

Step One Sample Menus

Day One
7:30 a.m.: Wake up
8:00 a.m. Breakfast:
> egg omelet with chopped bell peppers, onions, and tomato; 1 slice of
> low-carb toast (5-gram Counter Carb) with whipped butter and carb-
> free jelly; coffee with half-and-half and, if desired, erythritol, stevia,
> or Splenda

11:00 a.m. Midmorning snack:
> handful of almonds and 1 low-fat string cheese; 16 ounces of flavored
> water

1:45 p.m. Lunch:
> 1 low-carb wrap (5-gram Counter Carb) filled with sliced oven-baked
> turkey breast, low-fat cheese, shredded lettuce, tomato, and light
> mayonnaise; sugar-free gelatin; 16 ounces of water with lemon

4:00 p.m. Afternoon snack:
> strawberry protein shake (1 gram net carb); celery sticks with natural
> peanut butter

7:30 p.m. Dinner:
> generous piece of All-Veggie Lasagna (recipe on page 313); tossed
> salad with balsamic vinaigrette; Lemon Ricotta Pudding (recipe on
> page 336); 16 ounces of green tea

11:00 p.m. Bedtime snack:
> glass of unsweetened chocolate almond milk and 1 square of a
> graham cracker (5-gram Counter Carb)

Day Two

6:00 a.m. Wake up:
    vanilla protein shake (1 gram net carb)

7:00 a.m.
    Thirty minutes exercise

8:30 a.m. Breakfast:
    1 individual toaster-oven "pizza": low-carb tortilla (5-gram Counter
    Carb) with no-sugar-added marinara sauce, shredded low-fat
    mozzarella cheese, and a sprinkle of Parmesan; green tea
    (2 tea bags)

11:30 a.m. Midmorning snack:
    spoonful of natural peanut butter with celery sticks; coffee with
    half-and-half and, if desired, erythritol, stevia, or Splenda

1:30 p.m. Lunch:
    chicken soup (ordered as Chinese take-out) with a sprinkle of carrots
    and scallions—no noodles or rice (homemade chicken soup would
    be neutral, but a Chinese restaurant may use a carb-containing
    thickening agent; count Chinese chicken soup as a 5-gram Counter
    Carb: steamed shrimp and vegetables with no sauce—use some of
    the soup as "sauce"; ice water with lemon

4:30 p.m. Afternoon snack:
    low-fat string cheese and a handful of almonds; 16 ounces of water

7:30 p.m. Dinner:
    5 ounces of pinot grigio; grilled chicken; steamed broccoli with a dab
    of whipped butter; "Faux" Mashed Potatoes (recipe on page 318);
    sugar-free gelatin with light whipped cream

10:30 p.m. Bedtime snack:
    Chocolate Ricotta Pudding (recipe on page 335)

Breakfast Ideas for Step One

Egg-white omelet with peppers, onions, tomato, and mushrooms
(you may also consider regular whole eggs or egg substitute)
1 slice of low-carb toast (5-gram Counter Carb) with whipped butter

4 ounces of vegetable juice (neutral vegetable)
1 scoop of low-fat cottage cheese or part-skim ricotta cheese over
Romaine lettuce, carrot sticks, and bell pepper sticks

Low-carb chocolate protein shake (5-gram Counter Carb)
Handful of peanuts

Easy Egg Cups (recipe on page 261)
1 slice of Canadian bacon
1 slice of low-carb toast (5-gram Counter Carb) with natural almond
butter

8 ounces of unsweetened vanilla almond milk smoothie with ¼ cup
of low-carb protein shake, ¼ cup of unsweetened Greek yogurt,
⅓ cup of blueberries, stevia or Splenda to taste, and ½ cup of ice
(5-gram Counter Carb)
1 slice of toasted low-carb bread (5-gram Counter carb) with melted
cheese and tomato slices

Low-carb tortilla wrap (5-gram Counter Carb) spread with natural
peanut butter

Breakfast calzone: low-carb tortilla wrap (5-gram Counter Carb)
filled with lean ham and low-fat ricotta cheese, rolled, and heated
in toaster oven.

Low-carb yogurt (5 or fewer grams net carb)
Celery sticks with natural peanut butter

Miracle Quiche (recipe on page 263)
Zucchini Muffin (neutral) (recipe on page 332)

6 Silver Dollar Pancakes (recipe on page 269) with whipped butter and carb-free syrup
2 strips of turkey bacon

1 slice of low-carb toast (5 or fewer grams carb) with 1 tablespoon of natural peanut butter
1 cup of unsweetened chocolate soy or almond milk

1 slice of low-carb toast (5 or fewer grams carb) spread with low-fat ricotta cheese and cinnamon; heat in a toaster oven until warm

Lunch Ideas for Step One

Tuna salad with light mayonnaise on a bed of crisp lettuce and tomato wedges
Sugar-free gelatin

Veggie Couscous Soup (page 287)
Chicken Caesar salad without croutons and with Caesar dressing on the side (use sparingly)

Chef's salad with ham, cheese, egg, turkey, and low-fat cheese, with light dressing on the side
Cheesy Chips (recipe on page 227)

Sirloin burger without the bun, with low-carb ketchup (5-gram Counter Carb) and lettuce, tomato, and onion as desired
Roasted veggies

Miracle Grilled Cheese (recipe on page 281)
Tomato wedges
Chocolate Brownie Muffin (recipe on page 330)

Turkey and light cheese roll-ups with peppers and tomatoes, wrapped in a low-carb tortilla wrap (5 or fewer grams net carb)
2 Easy Snickerdoodles (recipe on page 336)

Low-carb yogurt (5 or fewer grams net carb)
Ham and cheese roll-ups
Celery sticks with peanut butter

Light cottage cheese in a hollowed red bell pepper "cup"
Tossed salad with balsamic vinaigrette
1 slice of low-carb toast spread with garlic butter (5-gram Counter
    Carb)

Grilled chicken strips over Romaine lettuce leaves sprinkled with
    feta cheese and almonds
Light dressing
Cheesy Chips (recipe on page 277)

Veggie Couscous Soup (recipe on page 287)
Turkey/cheese roll-ups
Cheddar Flax Crackers (recipe on page 326)

Chunky Chicken Salad (recipe on page 292) and ¼ cup of
    sun-dried tomatoes on a crisp salad base, with low-fat dressing
    of choice
Cheddar Flax Crackers (recipe on page 326)

1 slice of low-carb bread (5 or fewer grams net carb) with natural
    peanut butter and sugar-free jelly
Celery sticks with cream cheese
1 gram net carb low-carb protein shake (neutral)

Easy Pizza (recipe on page 266)
Antipasti: ham, fresh mozzarella, black olives, and tomatoes

Dinner Ideas for Step One

Spicy Shrimp and Zucchini served over Spaghetti Squash
    "Spaghetti" (recipes on pages 301 and 303)
Cranberry Walnut Cookies (recipe on page 337)

Roasted chicken breast with fat-free gravy (5-gram Counter Carb)
"Faux" Mashed Potatoes (recipe on page 318)
Green beans with almonds

London broil steak with sautéed mushrooms
1 slice of low-carb garlic toast (5-gram Counter Carb)
Broccoli with light cheese sauce

Broiled flounder
Oven-roasted peppers, onions, and zucchini
Cauliflower Rice (recipe on page 321)
Easy Snickerdoodles (recipe on page 336)

Spaghetti Squash "Spaghetti" (recipe on page 303)
1 slice of low-carb garlic bread (5 or fewer grams net carb)
Caesar salad with light dressing

Chicken Paprikash (recipe on page 302)
Steamed green beans
Chocolate Brownie Muffin (recipe on page 330) with light whipped
    cream topping

Tender Spinach Salad (recipe on page 290)
Handful of Cheesy Chips (recipe on page 277)
Cinnamon Ricotta Pudding (recipe on page 335)

Sliced turkey breast with low-fat gravy (5-gram Counter Carb)
"Faux" Mashed Potatoes (recipe on page 318)
Fresh steamed green beans with slivered almonds
Cinnamon Muffin (recipe on page 331)

Pork tenderloin
Roasted vegetables
Tossed salad with light dressing
No-sugar-added pudding (5 or fewer grams net carb)

Sirloin burger on a grilled Portobello mushroom (as a bun), with low-fat cheese, low-carb ketchup, and lettuce, tomato, and onion

Raw neutral vegetables with low-fat onion dip

Broiled cod
Broiled tomatoes with Parmesan cheese
Steamed spinach
Sugar-free gelatin with whipped topping

Turkey hot dogs with mustard in a low-carb wrap (5-gram Counter Carb)
Sweet-and-Sour Cucumbers (recipe on page 276)
Cheesy Chips (recipe on page 277)

Veggie or meatless burger (neutral if it contains 5 or fewer grams net carb) and light cheese, open faced on one slice of low-carb bread (5-gram Counter Carb) with low-carb ketchup
Dill pickle spears
Miracle Coleslaw (recipe on page 286)

Grilled pork chop
"Faux" Mashed Potatoes (recipe on page 318)
Asparagus tips

Baked chicken breast
Roasted eggplant, onions, mushrooms, peppers
Square of dark chocolate (5-gram Counter Carb)

Snack Ideas for Step One

Many people choose to use noncarb snacks and save their 5-gram counter Carbs for mealtime and their bedtime snack. Remember to avoid stacking carbs during Step One—you have the option to choose up to 5 grams of net carb at a meal or bedtime snack if meals are more than four to five hours apart or if the bedtime snack is more than two hours after dinner.

celery sticks with natural peanut butter or light cream cheese

Cheesy Chips (recipe on page 277) with salsa

Chocolate Brownie Muffin (recipe on page 330)

Cinnamon Muffin (recipe on page 331)

Crispy Tortilla Chips (recipe on page 276; 5-gram Counter Carb)

leftover protein and veggies from a previous meal

light-cheese wedges

low-carb shake (5-gram Counter Carb if it contains 2 to 5 grams net carb)

low-fat cottage cheese

Chocolate Meringue Cookies (recipe on page 338)

nuts (3 handfuls/day maximum)

olives

other neutral recipes (many can be found on www.miracle-ville.com)

part-skim string cheese

protein shake (5-gram Counter Carb if it contains 2 to 5 grams net carb)

Ricotta Puddings (recipes on pages 335–336)

spoonful of natural nut butter (no added sugar)

sugar-free gelatin with whipped topping

turkey or ham and cheese roll-ups

veggies with light dip

Zucchini Muffin (recipe on page 332)

It's Greek to Me!

Greek yogurt is thicker and creamier than regular yogurt and is a great yogurt choice for those with Met B. Finding a yogurt these days is a true project, as yogurts have added fiber, nuts, jellied fruit, and granola and come in fat-free, light, or full fat options—what to do?

Look for a yogurt with live cultures. Plain Greek yogurt has almost half the carbohydrate grams and half the sodium of regular plain yogurt. (The process of making Greek yogurt strains out more lactose [milk sugar] and liquid, resulting in a thicker, more protein-rich product— great for those with Met B.)

When fruit, granola, flavorings are added to any yogurt, the carb content increases. A two-third cup of plain yogurt may contain 6 grams net carb, whereas an equivalent amount of light, fruited Greek yogurt may contain 10 grams net carb. Always read the Nutrition Facts label.

Greek yogurt does not curdle when cooked, so it is easily used in cooking and can also be used as a replacement for sour cream or mayonnaise in salad dressings and as a heavy cream replacement.

A scant two tablespoons of plain Greek yogurt is considered neutral on MM.

Step One: Frequently Asked Questions

I am a compulsive "weigher," and I get on the scale every day—several times a day! I'm sticking to Step One like it's my job, but there has been no weight loss after seven days! In fact, on the first three days of the program I gained some weight. What the heck is going on?

Before you begin the Metabolism Miracle take your starting weight and *all* of the recommended body measurements (see Chapter 10). Look in Chapter 10, page 205, to find your expected weight/inch loss after your eight weeks, plus time added for slipups. Keep your records in a safe place, and don't step back on the scale until after the eighth week, with time added for slip-ups.

Weighing yourself daily or even weekly on MM shows nothing meaningful.

Keep in mind that this program not only brings about permanent weight loss but also cleans up the initial excesses in fats and glucose circulating in your blood as it rests your pancreas and liver. Only after the fifth day, when your liver has emptied its glycogen stores, will you begin burning excess fat; seven days is too soon to see a change in weight. Also, if you begin the program with significant excesses in glucose, cholesterol, and triglycerides, it may take longer than a week to start to lose your excess body fat.

Follow the plan, get physically active, take one day at a time, and measure your progress *after* eight weeks. The results will be worth the wait!

For the past eight weeks everyone has remarked that I look great. I feel rested and energized, and I've tightened my belt three holes. Well, I weighed myself after eight weeks. I lost within my target range of six to thirteen pounds—losing ten pounds. Why does it look as if I've lost twenty pounds?

On every other diet plan you lose a combination of water, fat, and muscle. Steps One and Two of the Metabolism Miracle are fat-burning phases. Body fat is light, fluffy, big-volume tissue, whereas muscle tissue and fluid is heavy. When you lose ten pounds of fat, it looks and feels like twenty.

MM retains what your body needs—muscle and water balance—and burns excess fat. Your clothes will fit as if you've lost twice the amount, and your lipids, blood pressure, and blood glucose will improve as if you've lost double the scale weight. Celebrate your loss and look forward to more!

It's been ten days since I began Step One, and I still have my "starter symptoms." What gives?

- You may be "stacking" 5-gram Counter Carbs. Remember that you have the *option* to have a 5-gram Counter Carb at breakfast, lunch, dinner, bedtime, and in the middle of the night if you are awake. These 5-gram Counter Carbs should not be closer than three hours apart, except for the bedtime 5-gram Counter Carb that can be used if more than two hours have passed since dinner.
- Your low-carb bread or other 5-gram Counter Carb choice may be "bogus," with inaccurate presentation of Nutrition Facts based on their ingredient list.
- You may be "undereating" neutral foods. Use lean protein, heart-healthy fat, and neutral veggies liberally.
- You may have an inadequate intake of water and decaffeinated beverages. Being slightly dehydrated can prolong the five-day "kicker." If you are five-foot-three or taller, you require a minimum of sixty-four ounces of water per day. Those under five-foot-three require a minimum of forty-eight ounces per day.
- Perhaps you are not exercising adequately. MM requires a minimum of thirty minutes of activity over and above your usual activity, five days per week. (See Chapter 9 for more.)
- Are you skipping vitamins/supplements? Chapter 8 has a list of recommended vitamins, minerals, and supplements. They will balance your Step One and help you feel your best.

Depending on your degree of excess insulin production, your starting blood glucose, Hb A1C, lipid levels, or carb intake prior to beginning MM, you may feel the "kick" more than others. But after a maximum of ten days on Step One you should have *no* starter symptoms.

Perhaps you are waiting to eat more than one hour in the morning and not taking your nighttime snack within one hour of bedtime. You should not go over four to five hours without eating a meal or snack. When you exceed five hours to eat, wait more than one hour after waking up before eating, or eat your last snack more than one hour before bedtime, you will slow your metabolic rate and slow your body's conversion to "fat burning."

I made it to four weeks on Step One and then caved at a friend's wedding. I had potatoes at dinner plus a piece of wedding cake. What now?

Get back on track ASAP. The longer you wait to get back in the saddle, the harder it will be to restart.

On Step One, for slip-ups that occur in one five-hour block of time, you will add three days to the end of your Step One. If you have excess carbohydrate in the morning, afternoon, and evening, count that as three slip-ups and add nine days to the end of your Step One.

Take note: every time you deviate from Step One you will upset your resting pancreas and liver. It takes three whole days to make up for each slip-up. Excess carbohydrate greatly upsets your body, insulin release, glycogen release, and fat storage. Remain true to Step One, and you'll be ready to move forward in eight weeks with no extra time for slip-ups.

Also, expect to feel symptoms of uncontrolled Met B after a slip-up. You may feel fatigue, crankiness, intense carb cravings, irritability, and melancholy after slip-ups on Step One. Don't get caught in this web and give in—get right back on Step One after a slip-up and don't deviate, or else you will begin to back slide.

I'm constipated during Step One. Help!

If you are constipated, it's probably due to inadequate fluid intake. It is possible you are not drinking the sixty-four ounces of water or caffeine-free fluid each and every day.

In Steps One and Two, both fat-burning phases, your kidneys must cleanse your bloodstream of the breakdown products from fat, and your body must flush this waste out with urine. If you don't drink an adequate amount of fluid, your body will take needed fluid from your tissues and even your gastrointestinal tract, and you will be left with hardened, difficult-to-pass stools. Even if you aren't thirsty, you must drink, drink, and drink!

Also be sure to keep up your fiber intake with raw vegetables, salads, nuts, and 5-gram Counter Carb whole-grain bread products. Two teaspoons of a fiber supplement powder, made of powdered plant fiber, can add 10 grams of fiber with no extra carb. Make certain to drink more water or decaf when you take a fiber supplement.

The other factor is getting a minimum of thirty minutes of exercise, five days a week. Exercising your muscles will also exercise your GI tract and enable you to keep things moving along.

I can't exercise on Step One. I get light-headed and weak, and my muscles ache afterward. What will happen if I do the diet portion but skip the exercise?

Although we place a great deal of emphasis on the three diet steps of the Metabolism Miracle, always remember that exercise is half the program. If you follow the diet but don't exercise, you will burn fat *and* muscle. MM, with diet and exercise, is designed to be a fat-burning program. We want to retain and tone our muscles, not lose them. Not only do muscles give us strength and tone; our active tissues also burn blood glucose for fuel.

After the first five days of Step One the liver and muscles are purposely rendered low on glycogen stores. If you exercise more than forty minutes on Step One, you will most likely feel winded, exhausted, and ravenously hungry, and your muscles might ache. Plan on exercising for forty minutes, and you can and should Fuel Forward (FF). For more on exercise and Fueling Forward, see Chapter 9.

I found a pudding with packaging that read, "Sugar-Free and Low in Carb." Sounds perfect for a Step One 5-gram Counter Carb. How can I be sure?

There is only one way to determine whether a food is allowed as a 5-gram Counter Carb on Step One of MM: check the Nutrition Facts label and use the net carb formula:

Total carb grams – dietary fiber grams = net carb grams

If a serving has 1 gram or less, it is neutral, in that serving size, for Step One.

If a serving's net carb is 2 to 6 grams (inclusive), it can be used as a 5-gram Counter Carb in that serving size.

The maximum net carb grams for a 5-gram Counter Carb for Step One is 6 grams net carb.

If a serving's net carb is over 6 grams, it is not appropriate as a 5-gram Counter Carb for Step One of MM.

Can I save all my 5-gram Counter Carbs and treat myself to 20 grams of net carb with dinner?

No. Make sure you space your 5-gram Counter Carbs by four to five hours. If you have them sooner, they stack, and this will cause your pancreas to over-release insulin and your liver to over-release glucagon. If you don't have the 5-gram Counter Carb in one five-hour period, you've lost those 5 grams.

Remember that you don't have to count carb grams for most of the lean protein, neutral vegetable, or healthy fat choices (page 60).

I have type 2 diabetes, take oral medication for blood glucose, and have been maintaining a fasting blood glucose of 200 mg/dL (11.1 mmol/L). Two weeks into Step One I felt a little shaky, dizzy, and sweaty, but when I checked my blood sugar, it was normal—for the first time in years. Why am I feeling as if I'm hypoglycemic when my actual blood glucose is normal?

Anyone who takes medication to lower blood glucose, either oral medication or insulin, should inform their physician *before* beginning MM because Step One *quickly* improves blood glucose. Because your blood sugar has been out of control for a while, your brain has come to accept that 200 mg/dL or more is a normal reading. This high blood glucose has become

WALKING ON SUNSHINE

I've become a fan of fifteen to thirty minutes of sunlight exposure per day. Many don't realize the sun helps activate vitamin D in the body. And the millions of people with uncontrolled Met B are already at a higher risk of vitamin D deficiency. When Met B folks stay out of the sun, vitamin D levels drop even lower! And we now know vitamin D deficiency is directly linked to obesity.

With the push for sunscreen and covering up from the sun to help protect from developing skin cancer, there seems to be a negative association linked to sunshine. Consider getting your sunshine earlier in the day and limit it to thirty minutes per day.

your own personal norm. When the Metabolism Miracle normalizes your blood glucose, your brain registers a lower than normal blood glucose, and you have symptoms of hypoglycemia even though your blood glucose is actually normal. After a few days pass with normalized blood glucose, your body and brain will realign with a new norm—a healthy norm. But as long as your blood glucose is in the normal range (over 70 mg/dL [3.9 mmol/L]), you do not need to treat it. Sit down, sip some water, and relax, and the feeling will pass.

If you do not take medication for diabetes (oral medication or insulin), you will not become hypoglycemic on this program. If you start the program while taking medication to reduce blood glucose and your number drops below 70 mg/dL (3.9 mmol/L), you have true hypoglycemia and must immediately treat the condition (see Chapter 12). Be sure to report low blood sugar readings as soon as possible to your doctor so he or she may decrease your medication's dosage and you can continue right along with Step One at a lower dose of medication.

Can I eat as much as I want of the neutral foods on Step One?

Foods in the lean protein, healthy fat, and neutral veggie list are low enough in carbohydrate grams to be considered neutral. Don't lose sight of the fact that protein and fat do contain calories. For example, one cup of natural peanut butter contains about sixteen hundred calories! Your body processes excess fat calories from the food you eat before it processes the fat on your body.

If you have a sensible snack of unsweetened, natural peanut butter, as in a spoonful or two, you are just fine. Lean protein and veggies are lower in fat and calories than natural peanut butter. If you are hungry, there's no problem with having six to eight ounces of lean protein at dinner. Huge portions, however, will slow your weight loss. If you are hungry at any time, eat! Just make sure the foods you choose are from the approved neutral food lists, and consume a reasonable portion.

I've finished my eight weeks (plus days added for slip-ups) on Step One. I have had excellent results—my weight and inches are within my target range for these eight weeks). Do I have to move to Step Two, as I "completed" Step One with excellent results? What will happen if I remain on Step One for another eight weeks?

Other low-carb programs have no specific plan to reintroduce dense carbohydrates. As a result, as soon as dieters move onto the next phase, step, or stage, they quickly begin to regain all their lost weight. As a result of failing to bring carbohydrates back to their diet without rapid regain and going off the tracks, many of these dieters choose to remain in the most restrictive stage of the diet to avoid this risk.

Those living the Metabolism Miracle program need not stay on Step One, fearing they can't move forward without weight regain. *After successfully completing* any eight-week block of Step One, including time for slip-ups, there are two choices: stay on Step One or move on to Step Two. When you move to Step Two of the Metabolism Miracle program dense carbs will re-enter your meals and snacks in a very methodical way. Carbohydrate choices must be of the right type, in the right amount, and at the right time interval. Yes, you can have your carbs and eat them too— *and* continue burning fat!

However, with a liberal intake of vegetables; lean protein; healthy fat; 5-gram Counter carbs; exercise; the use of vitamins, minerals, and supplements; increased fiber; and recommended water and decaffeinated beverages, you can safely remain on Step One for as long as you desire.

If, despite thinking you did a good job on Step One, your weight and inches do not match your expected range, take a moment to analyze the situation. Don't move forward until you find the reason your weight/inches did not fall into your expected weight/inch zone.

To make your own assessment, keep a two-day food log of how you followed Step One. Be honest with your critique so you can find the reason.

- You may have exceeded the carb limitations of Step One. (Step One is for neutral foods with the option of adding a 5-gram Counter Carb at meals and bedtime snack.)
- You might not have gotten sixty-four ounces of water or decaffeinated carb-free beverages daily. If you are under five-foot three, your water and decaffeinated fluid requirement is forty-eight ounces.
- You may have skipped meals and snacks or gone over five hours without eating.
- You may have exceeded one hour to eat after waking up in the morning.
- You may have gone to bed without having a snack within one hour of bedtime.
- You might be overeating proteins and fats.
- You may have failed to exercise over and above your usual physical activity for a minimum of thirty minutes, five times a week.
- You might not have taken the necessary vitamins and supplements.
- You may have unknowingly consumed bogus 5-gram Counter Carbs.

If you can't find significant errors in your food log, you can send your food log to me, Diane Kress, on www.Miracle-ville.com. It might be time to ask your physician to test your TSH (thyroid stimulating hormone) level. If your TSH is higher than normal, you may have hypothyroidism (slow metabolism caused by inadequate thyroid hormone) and require thyroid medication like Synthroid™ or Levoxyl™.

If you go through two cycles of Step One and have made necessary corrections to your program and still do not lose pounds and inches within your expected range, you may need to ask your MD about the medication metformin (see page 142–143).

Don't move forward to Step Two until you have found the problem with your Step One and taken the steps to correct it. If you know you did not do a clean Step One, it is in your best interest to reweigh, remeasure, check your expected weight/inch target, and redo Step One. You will get your deserved loss and move forward to Step Two the right way.

Step One for the Long Haul

I have worked with clients, patients, and readers who absolutely *love* Step One. They use the appropriate portions of dense carbs as their 5-gram Counter Carbs, and they don't want to move forward to Steps Two or Three.

For these program followers I recommend they follow all components of Step One, especially the vitamins and supplements, and remind them of the following tweaks that allow Step One for the long haul.

If you stay for long periods on Step One, you can take one meal "off" every two weeks (twice a month) and make up for it at the end of your eight weeks.

This twice-a-month "planned slip-up" will set your program back twelve days per eight weeks in terms of weight and inches lost, but it allows you to take a five-hour block "off" for weddings, parties, and celebrations without guilt. (Remember, when on Step One you must add three days for each slip-up, and this rule allows for four slip-ups in eight weeks.)

If you are going to be living on Step One for the long haul and choose to have one planned slip-up every two weeks, you will have slipped up two times in one month but four times over an eight-week period. Four slip-ups, with three days per slip-up, adds twelve days to the end of the "long haul" Step One.

So if you are following Step One for the long-haul with one slip-up every two weeks, you will reweigh at the eight-week mark, plus time added for other slip-ups, plus twelve days. Once you ascertain that you have lost within your expected inches/pounds, you can continue your "long haul" Step One and reweigh/remeasure after the next eight weeks plus time added for slip-ups plus twelve days.

6

Step Two—Transition
A Healthy Path to Carbs

During your eight weeks or more on Step One you lost fat, inches, and unwanted pounds. You stopped your carb cravings and are now in control and feel more energized than you have felt in years. You look and feel younger and have completed your metabolism's Step One housecleaning.

Although you can feel and see the benefits of Step One, it helps to understand the internal changes that occurred when you retuned your metabolism. Your previously overactive pancreas has rested and has not been over-releasing insulin for at least eight weeks. Your liver has significantly decreased glycogen release.

Once you completed the first five days of Step One you stepped into a fat-burning zone, releasing less insulin and less glycogen and stabilizing your blood glucose.

Your blood lipids (cholesterol and triglycerides) and blood pressure markedly improved. Your fat cells began to shrink, and your insulin keys now fit the receptors on your cells. In short, your Metabolism B is now under control.

Step Two reintroduces healthy portions of low-impact carbohydrate foods at specific times so you will maintain fat burning with your liver and pancreas working in a normal fashion.

Lean protein, healthy fat, and neutral veggies remain neutral on Step Two. In addition to the neutral foods you will purposely add servings of mild carbohydrate chosen from a long list of low-impact carb foods.

These foods will enable your pancreas to gently reawaken, preventing it from overreacting with excessive insulin release.

Step Two is a nutritionally balanced way of eating that allows for safe, long-term weight loss. Plan to stay on Step Two for at least eight weeks or even remain on Step Two until you reach your desired weight or size. There is no limit to the amount of time you may stay on Step Two.

You may also alternate eight-week blocks of Step One and Step Two until you reach your desired size and weight. But when you do reach your desired weight and size make sure you finish Step Two before moving on to Step Three. Each step transitions into the next, so they must be done in this order.

How Step Two Works

Let's take a peek inside your body to understand what happens when you reintroduce carbohydrate in Step Two.

For the past eight-plus weeks on Step One your liver's glycogen stores were purposely depleted. After the first five days of Step One the liver

began a vacation from "self-feeding" for the remainder of Step One. Instead of burning glucose from carbohydrate foods or the liver's release of
glycogen stores, your body went into fat-burning mode.

On the morning you begin Step Two the right amount of low-impact
carbohydrate will gently enter your bloodstream at regular intervals.
Throughout Step Two the idea is to begin feeding your metabolism one
11- to 20-gram net Carb Dam within an hour of waking up and within one
hour of bedtime. Build an 11- to 20-gram Carb Dam at breakfast (within
one hour of waking up), lunch, dinner, bedtime snack (within one hour of
going to bed), *and* anytime you have more than five hours between your
meals. Your body will become accustomed to having appropriate mild
carbs in a set amount (11 to 20 grams net carb) at appropriate intervals
from morning until bedtime.

By fueling your body in this way you will not rely on the liver's release
of glycogen stores while you are awake. With this purposeful regularity
of carb consumption your rested pancreas will release a normal amount
of insulin, and the liver will remain filled with glycogen. While you sleep
the liver will release glycogen stores at four- to five-hour intervals. This
will keep your blood sugar stable while you sleep.

Step Two's methodical feeding schedule allows your liver to gradually refill with glycogen and resume its job of *back-up* glucose provider.
From the first day of Step Two, if you wait more than four to five hours

without eating an 11- to 20-gram Carb Dam, your liver will automatically release glycogen stores. And your liver, in its self-feed mode, will release far more than 11 to 20 grams of carbohydrate. I estimate that the liver releases 45 to 65 grams net carb (glycogen) when more than five hours pass between meals. That's a whole lot more than our extra 11- to 20-gram Carb Dam snack between distant meals. In other words, failing to have an 11- to 20-gram between-meal snack will open the door for a deposit of about 45 to 65 grams from the liver!

The more often the liver is called upon to dispense glycogen, the more frequently your blood sugar will spike and the more taxed your pancreas becomes. In short order your pancreas returns to insulin imbalance, expanding fat cells, and insulin resistance—uncontrolled Met B.

Step Two is specifically designed to prevent this return to metabolic chaos. By introducing a specific type of mild carbohydrate in a very specific amount (11 to 20 net grams) at the right time (meals no more than five hours apart unless there is an 11- to 20-gram snack between the meals), you will retain control over your blood glucose and insulin as you continue to lose weight and inches and love the way you look and feel.

Step Two: A Switch-Up in Your Program

After the fifth day of Step One your liver was purposely depleted of major glycogen stores. As you curtailed your carbohydrate intake, the liver could not overcontribute in its self-feeding mode. The focus on lean protein, heart-healthy fat, and neutral veggies kept your dense carbohydrate intake at a low level so your body would burn fat. Step One is a minimalist phase with a goal of preventing sharp spikes and drops in blood glucose. Step Two, in contrast, shows you how to consume a safe amount of mild carbohydrate at the right intervals and still remain in fat-burning mode.

The Carb Dam: 11 to 20 Grams Net Carb Is the Magic Number

The 11 to 20 grams of net carb is the amount of net carbohydrate small enough to prevent overstimulating the pancreas yet high enough to prevent the liver from engaging in self-feeding. This carb gram range means business! All 11- to 20-gram Carb Dams should come from the lists of low-impact carbs (page 122).

Time your carbohydrates in the correct portions throughout the day, and you have effectively set up a dam that prevents the liver from releasing glycogen. It is critical to keep the amount of carbohydrate between 11 and 20 grams *inclusive*. On Step Two you *must have* an 11- to 20-gram Carb Dam at meals, bedtime, and when time between meals exceeds five hours. There is no "stacking" on Step Two; your 11- to 20-gram Carb Dams are *necessary* to keep your liver from releasing glycogen. These 11- to 20-gram Carb Dams are *not* optional; they are necessities because they block the liver from being called upon for glycogen release.

A dam built of fewer than 11 grams net carb will not be high enough to prevent liver glycogen from flowing over. A dam built of more than

20 grams of carbohydrate at a meal or snack will cause blood sugar to quickly rise and stimulate the pancreas to release extra insulin, which will lead to fat gain rather than fat loss.

Don't fear Carb Dams on Step Two, as they are your new "medication." The 11 to 20 grams of net carb from the low-impact lists is able to stop your liver from over-releasing glycogen stores and ruining your wonderful progress.

These 11 to 20 grams of low-impact carb properly placed is what Step Two is all about. Proper carb placement enables the pancreas and liver to awaken gently and keep you in weight-loss mode. *Missing a Carb Dam is a slip-up on Step Two.*

The Trusty Net Carb Gram Formula (with a Twist)

So how do you keep your carbohydrate grams within the 11- to 20-gram range? Page 122 provides lists of approved Step Two carb choices. But how will you know if a prepackaged starchy carbohydrate choice, like cereal, crackers, bars, or bread, makes the grade as a *mild* carb?

In Step Two do the trusty net carb formula as you would during Step One, but after you ascertain the serving size has 11 to 20 grams net carb, take a quick look at *fiber* and *sugar* for *starchy* foods only. Do not check the label of packaged fruit like jarred peaches, milk, pudding, or yogurt for fiber content or sugar grams. The Step Two fiber and sugar gram rule is *not* used when choosing packaged fruit or milk products. For these foods just make sure the amount you are going to consume has 11 to 20 grams net carb, inclusive.

If the starchy food choice has 11 to 20 grams net carb and the right amount of fiber and sugar, it's a great Carb Dam. To qualify as mild, the rule for packaged starches with 11 to 20 grams net carb is:

On Step Two

Net carb grams must be between 11 and 20 grams, inclusive.
Dietary fiber needs to be 2 grams or more.
Sugar grams need to be 6 grams or fewer.

You already know how to use the net carb formula from Step One:

Total carbohydrate grams – dietary fiber grams = net carb grams

In Step Two you'll use the same formula to guarantee that starch-based packaged foods such as bread, crackers, cereal, bars, and snack products are within the 11- to 20-gram window *and* are considered mild carb grams. First, check the Nutrition Facts label and plug the numbers into your trusty formula.

Light Whole-Grain Bread

Serving Size 2 slices

Total Carbohydrate 20 grams

Dietary Fiber 3 grams

Sugar 1 gram

20 – 3 = 17 net carb grams

Two slices of this bread fit into the 11- to 20-gram window, so now you need to double-check on dietary fiber grams and sugar grams.

The two slices of Light Whole-Wheat Bread have 17 grams net carb (good), dietary fiber of 3 grams (good), and sugar grams of 1 gram (good). So on all three counts this particular bread is a great choice as an 11- to 20-gram Carb Dam.

Let's try another. Is this an appropriate starchy food for an 11- to 20-gram Carb Dam?

Cinnamon Crunch Granola

Serving Size ¼ cup

Total Carbohydrate 23 grams

Dietary Fiber 4 grams

Sugar 9 grams

23 – 4 = 19 grams net carb

So the granola is in the 11- to 20-gram Carb Dam range, but is it mild enough? With its dietary fiber of 4 grams (good) but its sugar of 9 grams (excessive), a quarter-cup of Cinnamon Crunch Granola is *too high in sugar* for Step Two!

At lunch you decide to have some multigrain crackers with your chicken Caesar salad. How many crackers can you have and still be within the 11- to 20-gram target range with the right fiber and sugar content? Simply check the Nutrition Facts label.

Multigrain Crackers

Serving Size 8 crackers

Total Carbohydrate 24 grams

Dietary Fiber 5 grams

Sugar 2 grams

---

24 − 5 = 19 net carb grams

Eight crackers fit into the 11- 20-gram window, so go ahead and check fiber and sugar, as crackers are a starchy food choice. With the fiber at 5 grams (good) and the sugar at 2 grams (good), you can enjoy this product on Step Two!

For the next eight weeks you should choose all of your carb servings from the Low-Impact Carbs list (page 122). Whole-grain bread and multigrain crackers are on the list, but high-impact carbs such as marshmallows, potato chips, and oversweetened bars are not. Keep them out of Step Two to prevent yourself from backsliding.

Timing Is Everything

Once you enter Step Two you must not go longer than five hours without including an 11- to 20-gram Carb Dam, beginning within one hour of waking up and ending within one hour of going to bed. This timing of Carb Dams throughout the day will keep your metabolism stoked for higher fat burning. If you fail to keep your blood sugar at the status quo with 11- to 20-gram Carb Dams, your body will flip the switch on your liver to overcompensate with glycogen release. In turn, the pancreas will overreact with excess insulin, cravings will return, and you will regain fat and inches you had previously lost.

Remember that Step Two is properly reprogramming your metabolism to accept carb grams and continue to burn fat. You want to program it with the right amount of low-impact carbohydrate at the right time. This is a period of transition. If you skip the transition and introduce carbs haphazardly, you will most definitely regain everything you've lost.

To recap: during Step Two you must eat a mild 11- to 20-gram Carb Dam at the following times:

- within one hour of waking up
- prior to exercising first thing in the morning (if you exercise before breakfast)
- with breakfast, lunch, and dinner
- at snacks between meals that exceed five hours apart
- within one hour of going to sleep at night
- if you wake up during the middle of the night (optional but not required)

Choose all of your 11- to 20-gram Carb Dams from the Low-Impact Carbs list (page 122).

Keep Them Coming

It's hard to believe but, once you reintroduce carbs, you must keep them coming or else you will regain weight. It is very possible you'll need six or more carb servings of 11- to 20-gram Carb Dams per day, depending on your lifestyle.

Here's a typical day's carb placement for Step Two:

7:00 a.m.: Wake up
8:00 a.m.: Breakfast (11 to 20 grams net carb)
11:00 a.m.: Midmorning snack with 11 to 20 grams net carb (because breakfast and lunch are more than five hours apart)
1:30 p.m.: Lunch (11 to 20 grams net carb)
4:30 p.m.: Midafternoon snack with 11 to 20 grams net carb (lunch and dinner are more than five hours apart)

7:30 p.m.: Dinner (11 to 20 grams net carb)

10:30 p.m.: Bedtime snack (11 to 20 grams net carb)

11:00 p.m.: Bedtime

(For specific examples, see "Step Two Sample Menu" on page 126)

The First Five Days of Step Two

Most people notice a little bloating and tighter waistlines during the first five days of Step Two. Don't worry about this: relax and stay off the scale—you are not regaining fat!

As your liver and muscles refill with glycogen, additional fluid is retained. Drink plenty of water to help your body release this excess fluid retention. By the fifth day of Step Two the bloating will have disappeared and your waistband will be back to normal.

After those first five days your body should continue to feel healthy and energized. If you mistakenly hop on the scale during these first days, you may see weight gain from fluid retention. Learn Step Two as if it were your job; doing so will put you in control of your weight and health for life.

As with all of the Steps of the Metabolism Miracle, be sure to follow the ten Rules to Thrive By (page 172). Pay particular attention to *timing*, *drinking* at least sixty-four ounces of caffeine-free fluid daily, exercising a *minimum* of thirty minutes, five times a week, and taking the recommended *supplements*.

When you exercise thirty to sixty minutes on Step Two there is no need to Fuel Forward (see Chapter 9) because your liver is refilled with glycogen and will fuel your first hour of exercise. If, however, your exercise will last one and a half hours or more, begin Fueling Forward at the one-hour mark. This won't be necessary if you are taking a slow walk, but consider adding Fueling Forward in Step Two for a distance bike ride, marathon running, training for a marathon, or if your gym workout will last one and a half hours or more.

Step Two is a nutritionally balanced, fat-burning phase you can follow for as long as you like and continue to lose weight. Once you have reached the weight that you desire and achieve maximum health on as little medication as possible, step on the scale and check your weight.

The weight at which you are healthy and look and feel great is *your* desired body weight and size.

Low-Impact Carb Dams

Choose any low-impact Carb Dam from the following low-impact carbs list for your breakfast, lunch, dinner, and nighttime snack. If the time between meals exceeds five hours, place an *extra* carb serving of 11 to 20 grams mild net carbohydrate between them.

All portions shown are ready to eat and equal 11 to 20 grams net carbohydrate.

Step Two Carb Dams

For all carb servings listed in this section, one serving must contain 11 to 20 grams of net carb, 2 or more grams of fiber and 6 or fewer grams of sugar. Read your Nutrition Labels if you're not sure whether your Carb Dam choice meets these guidelines.

Breads (Starch)
    2 slices of thin-sliced, light, or lower-carb whole-grain bread
    1 slice of whole-grain bread
    1 light whole-grain English muffin
    ½ whole-grain English muffin
    1 light or lower-carb whole-grain pita
    ½ whole-grain pita
    1-ounce portion of bakery bread and rolls

Cereals and Grains
    ½ cup of cooked oatmeal
    ½ cup of cooked barley
    ½ cup of cooked brown or wild rice
    ½ cup of cooked whole-grain pasta (cooked al dente)
    ½ cup of cooked bulgur

½ cup of cooked quinoa
1 serving of dry cereal (2 grams or more of fiber and 6 grams or less of sugar)

Specialty or Bakery Breads
Give thin-sliced, light, and lower-carb breads a try. With half the carb grams of regular breads (one slice of whole-wheat bread has the same carb grams as two slices of light whole-wheat bread), they can allow you to have twice as much for your 11- to 20-net carb allotment. Both of these bread choices have 2 or more grams of fiber, 6 or fewer grams of sugar, and between 11 and 20 grams of net carb, making both choices perfect for Step Two. Fiber may be lower than 2 grams unless you purchase a hearty grain or multigrain with seeds bread.

Crackers and Starchy Snacks
1 serving of whole-grain crackers
3 cups of popcorn (light or hot air–popped, with no partially hydrogenated oils or trans fats)

1 serving of whole-grain pretzels
1 serving of tortilla chips

Protein Bars
Before snacking on a protein bar, be sure to read the Nutrition Label to make sure one serving contains 11 to 20 grams of net carb, 2 or more grams of fiber and 6 or fewer grams of sugar.

Starchy Vegetables and Legumes
½ cup of corn
½ ear of fresh corn
½ cup of peas
½ cup of legumes such as kidney beans, lentils, lima beans,
    chickpeas, white beans, black beans, or white kidney beans
⅓ cup of hummus
½ sweet potato or yam or ½ cup of mashed sweet potato or yam
1½ cups of cooked carrots or 1½ cups of raw carrots
1 cup of beets

Soups
1 cup of tomato soup (water based)
½ cup of lentil soup
½ cup of split-pea soup
1 cup of chicken noodle soup (whole-grain noodles or brown rice)
Any soup in an 11- to 20-gram carb serving with fiber greater than
    2 grams per serving

Fruit
All of the following portions represent 11 to 20 grams net carb. Fruit choices should be average in size.

1 apple (medium, 3-inch diameter)
1 pear (small, or ½ large pear)
1 peach (medium, or 3-inch diameter)
2 plums (medium, or 2⅛-inch diameter)
1 nectarine (medium, or 3-inch diameter)
⅔ cup of unsweetened natural applesauce

CEREAL FOR BREAKFAST?

Remember that both milk and cereal net carbs must total 11 to 20 grams to count as an 11- to 20-gram Carb Dam. A half cup of milk contains 6 grams of net carb. To help increase your serving of cereal, substitute unsweetened soy or almond milk for cow's milk, as these milk substitutes are neutral.

For example, three-fourths cup of cereal has 23 grams total carb, with 4 grams of fiber and 5 grams of sugar. So three-fourths cup of this cereal is an appropriate 11- to 20-gram Carb Dam, as it contains 11 to 20 grams net carb. With one-half cup of unsweetened almond or soy milk, which is neutral, the total carb count comes to 19 grams net carb.

½ grapefruit (4- to 5-inch diameter for full fruit; AVOID grapefruit if you are taking the statin Lipitor™)

15 medium or 12 large cherries

1 cup of sliced strawberries

1 cup of blackberries

1 cup of blueberries

1 cup of raspberries

2 clementine oranges or 2 small tangerines

4 apricots or 8 dried apricot halves

15 medium or 12 large grapes

1 orange

1 cup (4 ounces) pineapple cubes

½ medium banana

Milk, Yogurt*, Ice Cream, Pudding

Maintain the 11 to 20 grams net carb per serving, but you don't need to check fiber.

1 cup (8 fluid ounces) of fat-free, nonfat, 1%, 2%, or skim-plus milk

Plain or Greek yogurt*

1 cup (8 fluid ounces) of buttermilk

Fruit-flavored yogurt sweetened with Splenda or sucralose*

½ cup of sugar-free, fat-free pudding

FRUIT TIPS

Beware of Giant Fruit
When you choose fruit take stock of its size. You needn't buy the smallest apple in the basket, but the orange that looks more like a basketball isn't a good option either. Train your eye to focus on average or medium-sized fresh fruit that fits into the 11- to 20-gram net carb rule.

Just Say NO to Juice
With its high-impact carbohydrate and negligible fiber, fruit juice spikes your blood sugar like a rocket, causing the Met B pancreas to overreact. Fruit juice is never a good choice if you have Metabolism B unless you are using it as a treatment for hypoglycemia (see page 232).

Missing Your Favorite Fruit?
If a preferred fruit is absent from the Step Two fruit category, it probably isn't an oversight. The fruits included on this list are low impact and fit well into this transitional stage when you are being cautious with restarting your pancreas. Other fruits will come back into the picture when you enter Step Three.

No-sugar-added ice cream products sweetened with Splenda or
   erythritol

*If you are choosing a yogurt for Step Two, please use the yogurt rule in the box opposite.

Step Two Sample Menus

Remember, timing is critical. You should never go more than five hours without an 11- to 20-gram net carb serving in the form of another meal or snack. In the sample menu below each 11- to 20-gram net carb serving is noted.

DAIRY TIPS

Eight ounces of milk contain 11 to 20 grams of net carb, regardless of the milk's fat content. The benefit of consuming lower-fat versions is that they can help in a fat-burning weight-loss program.

Don't look at fiber and sugar grams on milk's Nutrition Facts; milk is fiber-free and most of the carbohydrate/sugar grams come from lactose (milk sugar).

The Yogurt Rule

While in Step Two it's important to choose the right yogurt. Although most of the sugar grams on yogurt's Nutrition Facts come from lactose (milk sugar), yogurt companies also add sugar to plain yogurt when they produce fruit or fruit-flavored yogurt. To make sure your yogurt is not overdoing it with the added sugar, here's an easy chart to help you make the right choice.

Ounces of yogurt	Net carb in this amount of yogurt from lactose	Added sugar limit for this amount of yogurt
8	12	No more than 18 grams total of sugar
6	9	No more than 15 grams total of sugar
5	7.5	No more than 13.5 grams total of sugar
4	6	No more than 12 grams total of sugar

Welcome Back, Ice Cream

Look for ice cream that has sucralose (brand name Splenda), stevia, or erythritol rather than sugar or aspartame as the primary sweetener. Even if the net carb appears the same in sugar-sweetened ice cream, the type of carbohydrate is very different from that in stevia-, Splenda-, and erythritol-sweetened products. Sugar-sweetened desserts are high-impact carbohydrates.

6:30 a.m. Wake up

8:00 a.m. Breakfast:
1 light multigrain English muffin (11- to 20-gram Carb Dam) with natural cashew butter and 2 teaspoons of carb-free jelly; coffee with half-and-half and, if desired, erythritol, stevia, or Splenda

10:00 a.m.:
Midmorning snack: string cheese (An 11- to 20-gram net Carb Dam is *not* needed because breakfast and lunch are *within* five hours.)

12:00 p.m. Lunch:
grilled cheese sandwich made with tomato slices and 2 slices of light whole-grain bread (11- to 20-gram Carb Dam); iced unsweetened green tea with lemon (add erythritol, stevia, or Splenda if desired)

4:00 p.m. Midafternoon snack:
dip of low-fat cottage cheese with 1 cup of strawberry halves (11- to 20-gram Carb Dam)

6:00 p.m. Dinner:
broiled flounder; ½ cup of cooked wild rice (11- to 20-gram Carb Dam); a lot of steamed broccoli; 1 Chocolate Brownie Muffin (neutral, recipe on page 330); decaf coffee with half-and-half and, if desired, erythritol, stevia, or Splenda

10:30 p.m. Nighttime snack:
1 serving of peach-flavored Greek Yogurt (11- to 20-gram Carb Dam)

Step Two Sample Menu

6:00 a.m.: Wake up

6:30 a.m.: Pre-exercise snack:
⅔ cup of unsweetened natural applesauce (11- to 20-gram Carb Dam), then exercise for forty-five minutes

8:00 a.m. Breakfast:

4 ounces tomato juice (neutral in this serving size); scrambled egg whites with 2 strips of turkey bacon; 2 slices of light multigrain toast (11- to 20-gram Carb Dam) with whipped butter; coffee with half-and-half and, if desired, erythritol, stevia, or Splenda. Because breakfast and lunch are within five hours of each other, you won't need a midmorning snack.

1:00 p.m. Lunch:

scoop of homemade chicken salad with light mayonnaise; Romaine lettuce and sliced tomato; 1 whole-grain wrap (11- to 20-gram Carb Dam size); ⅓ cup berries of any kind (5 grams net carb—when added to wrap, you are still in the 11- to 20-gram Carb Dam range)

4:00 p.m. Midafternoon snack:

1 gram net carb protein shake (neutral); handful of cashews (because lunch and dinner are within five hours of each other, an 11- to 20-gram Carb Dam is not necessary at this snack)

6:00 p.m. Dinner:

5 ounces merlot (neutral and approved by MD); homemade meatloaf made with 85% ground sirloin and Parmesan cheese in place of breadcrumbs; 2 tablespoons of low-fat gravy (neutral); ½ whipped sweet potato (11- to 20-gram Carb Dam); oven-roasted green beans; tea with lemon

11:00 p.m. Bedtime snack:

1 cup of low-fat milk (11–20 gram Carb Dam); 2 Chocolate Meringues (recipe on page 338)

Breakfast Suggestions for Step Two

Veggie omelet with low-fat cheese

1 light multigrain English muffin (11- to 20-gram Carb Dam) with natural unsweetened peanut butter and carb-free jelly

1 container of light, flavored Greek yogurt (9 grams net carb) and 7
  Wheat Thins crackers (7 grams net carb) to equal 11–20 gram Carb
  Dam

Grilled cheese: Made with 2 slices light multigrain bread (11- to
  20-gram Carb Dam), low-fat Cheddar cheese, tomato slices, and
  whipped butter

Whole grain cereal in an amount to equal an 11- to 20-gram Carb Dam
Unsweetened plain or flavored almond or soy milk (neutral)

Leftover protein from last night's dinner
1 low carb wrap (5 grams net carb) plus 1 cup cantaloupe cubes (15
  grams net carb) to equal an 11- to 20-gram Carb Dam

½ cup of cooked oatmeal or 1 prepared envelope of unflavored
  cooked oatmeal (11- to 20-gram Carb Dam)
Sprinkle of cinnamon, walnuts, and Splenda, erythritol, or stevia, if
  desired

2 slices of thin-sliced whole-grain toast (11- to 20-gram Carb Dam)
Spread with carb -free jelly and natural unsweetened peanut butter
Unsweetened chocolate flavored soy or almond milk

Fruit Smoothie with a base of ½ cup of Greek Yogurt, 1 cup of mixed
  berries (11- to 20-gram Carb Dam) and ½ cup of unsweetened
  vanilla soy or almond milk, plus a scoop of low-carb whey protein
  powder; sweeten with Splenda, erythritol, or stevia to taste

Zucchini Muffin (recipe on page 332)
Scoop of Ricotta Pudding of your choice (recipes on pages 335–336)
15 grapes (11- to 20-gram Carb Dam)

Light cottage cheese or ricotta cheese (can be sweetened with
  erythritol, Splenda, or stevia)
1 cup of sliced strawberries (11- to 20-gram Carb Dam)

Sprinkling of sliced almonds

Neutral muffin (Cinnamon, Chocolate, or zucchini; recipes on pages 330–332)

1 toasted light multigrain English muffin (11- to 20-gram Carb Dam) topped with a sunny-side-up egg, Canadian bacon, and low-fat cheese. Microwave the sandwich to melt the cheese.

Lunch Suggestions for Step Two

Easy Pizza (recipe on page 266; 11- to 20-gram Carb Dam)

Chilled green tea with lemon

Tuna salad made with light mayonnaise atop a salad of dark lettuce, spring mix, or neutral salad of your choice, with pitted olives, avocado slices, cherry tomatoes, and balsamic vinaigrette

½ cup of chickpeas (11- to 20-gram Carb Dam)

Cheesy Chips (recipe on page 277)

Sandwich of 2 slices light whole-grain bread (11- to 20-gram Carb Dam), thinly sliced oven-roasted turkey breast, Lorraine Swiss, lettuce, tomato slices, and light mayonnaise

Burger (85 to 93 percent lean ground beef) with low-fat cheese on a multigrain burger bun (11- to 20-gram Carb Dam) with low-carb ketchup (e.g., Heinz™ reduced-sugar or Walden Farms™), lettuce, tomato, onion, and dill pickle slices

Cheesy Chips (recipe on page 277)

1 cup of tomato soup (11- to 20-gram Carb Dam)

Neutral salad with protein and dressing on the side (e.g., chicken Caesar with no croutons or chef's, Cobb, or steak salad)

6 ounces of light, fruit-flavored Greek yogurt (9 grams net carb) with ⅓ cup of fresh blueberries (together equaling an 11- to 20-gram Carb Dam)

Celery sticks with natural, unsweetened peanut butter

Stir-fried tofu sautéed in olive oil with lots of neutral veggies (e.g., chopped broccoli, 3 baby carrots, onion)
½ cup of fluffy brown rice (11- to 20-gram Carb Dam)

Deli sandwich on 2 slices of light multigrain bread (11–20 gram Carb Dam), shaved turkey or roast beef, low-fat Cheddar cheese, dark lettuce, tomato slices, and light mayonnaise
Dill pickle

Low-carb pita (11- to 20-gram Carb Dam) filled with grilled chicken breast strips, shredded lettuce, shredded cheese, tomato wedges, and light salad dressing

Chef's salad with cheese, turkey, ham, eggs, and light dressing
1 serving of whole-grain crackers (11- to 20-gram Carb Dam)

Philly Cheese Steak (recipe on page 305) on 1 light multigrain burger bun (11- to 20-gram Carb Dam) with sautéed peppers and onions
Miracle "Faux-Tato" Salad (recipe page 295)

Light cottage cheese or ricotta cheese
1 cup of sliced strawberries (11- to 20-gram Carb Dam)
Zucchini Muffin (recipe page 332)

Turkey, ham, cheese roll-ups
½ cup of Pasta Primavera Salad (recipe on page 293; 11- to 20-gram Carb Dam)

Dinner Suggestions for Step Two
Roasted turkey with low-fat gravy
"Faux" Mashed Potatoes (recipe on page 318)
½ cup of corn kernels (11- to 20-gram Carb Dam)
Chocolate Ricotta Pudding (recipe on page 335)

Grilled chicken breast or rotisserie chicken
Caesar salad without croutons

1 cup of sliced strawberries and whipped cream (11- to 20-gram Carb Dam)

Dish of Miracle Noodles™ or shirataki noodles with ½ cup of marinara sauce (no sugar added) with ground turkey and topped with grated Parmesan cheese
Garden salad with balsamic vinaigrette
1 ounce of whole-grain bakery bread made into garlic bread (11- to 20-gram Carb Dam)

Grilled lean steak
Sweet Potato Fries with "Maple Syrup" Dip (recipe page 319; 11- to 20-gram Carb Dam)
Miracle Coleslaw (recipe on page 286)
Chocolate Brownie Muffin (recipe on page 330)

Chicken cheese steak (with low-fat cheese) on 1 low-carb multigrain bun (11- to 20-gram Carb Dam) with grilled onions and bell peppers and reduced-sugar ketchup (e.g., Heinz or Walden Farms)
Side salad with vinaigrette dressing
2 Thumbprint Peanut Butter and Jelly Cookies (recipe on page 329)

Grilled pork chops
Cauliflower Rice (recipe on page 321)
Asparagus spears
⅔ cup of unsweetened natural applesauce (11- to 20-gram Carb Dam)

Chicken cutlets coated with grated Parmesan cheese in place of bread crumbs
8 Sweet Potato Fries with "Maple Syrup" Dip (recipe on page 319; 11- to 20-gram Carb Dam)
Miracle Coleslaw (recipe on page 286)
Sugar-free gelatin with whipped topping

Broiled flounder
"Faux" Mashed Potatoes (recipe on page 318)

Tender Spinach Salad (recipe on page 290)
Baked Apple (recipe on page 330; 11- to 20-gram Carb Dam)

Chicken Paprikash (recipe on page 302) served over ½ cup of whole-grain pasta (11- to 20-gram Carb Dam)
Sweet-and-Sour Cucumbers (recipe on page 276)
Sugar-free gelatin with whipped topping

Snack Suggestions for Step Two

Use these snacks only if an 11- to 20-gram Carb Dam snack is required. These snacks are to be used between meals in which the time between the start of one meal and the start of the next meal exceeds five hours. They can also be used for a bedtime snack when dinner and bedtime are two hours or more apart.

Whole-grain crackers (11 to 20 grams net carb) with natural unsweetened peanut butter or cheese
1 crisp apple, cut in wedges with a dip of natural peanut butter
Baked Apple (recipe on page 330)
1 cup of nonfat or 1% milk
1 serving of light yogurt (11 to 20 grams net carb)
5 to 6 ounces of light fruit-flavored Greek Yogurt with ⅓ serving of Step Two fruit (together equaling an 11- to 20-gram Carb Dam)
1 protein bar (fiber over 2 grams, sugar 6 or fewer grams, and 11 to 20 grams net carb)
3 cups of light popcorn (no trans or hydrogenated fats; 11 to 20 grams net carb)
½ cup of light ice cream sweetened with Splenda (11 to 20 grams net carb) and topped with nuts
¾ to 1 of cup cereal (fiber over 2 grams, sugar 6 or fewer grams, and 11 to 20 grams net carb) with unsweetened almond or soy milk
½ cup of cooked oatmeal (or 1 packet of unflavored oatmeal) with cinnamon, Splenda, slivered nuts, and unsweetened coconut flakes, if desired
½ cup of sugar-free pudding (11 to 20 grams net carb)

1 piece of Step Two fresh fruit

1 serving of whole-grain pretzels (11 to 20 grams net carb)

2/3 cup of unsweetened natural applesauce

8 dried apricot halves and a handful of nuts

Baked Apple (recipe on page 330)

Snack crackers (serving size with fiber over 2 grams, sugar 6 or fewer grams, and 11 to 20 grams net carb)

Step Two: Frequently Asked Questions

When I was on Atkins I regained all of my lost weight as soon as I added carbohydrate grams to my diet. How will I ever lose weight by adding carbohydrate back to my diet on Metabolism Miracle?

Unlike low-carb diets, MM is actually a carb-centric diet. The focus is always on carb grams. We choose lean protein, heart-healthy fats, and neutral veggies. Step Two reintroduces carbohydrate foods in a very methodical way—the right type of carbohydrate (low glycemic index and glycemic load) in the right amount at the right time (11 to 20 grams at each meal and at nighttime, with an additional 11 to 20 grams between meals that are more than five hours apart). Weigh and remeasure yourself before Step Two, find your expected loss after the next eight weeks, follow the program, and reweigh and remeasure at the end of the eighth week. You will be pleased to see your that weight and inch loss will be within your expected range.

I stepped on the scale four days into Step Two (I know I wasn't supposed to!), and I've gained weight! The waist on my jeans is tight, and I feel bloated. Should I return to Step One?

Did you end Step One by losing within your expected weight- and inch-loss zone? If so, you were ready to take on Step Two.

During the first five days of Step Two you will most likely not lose weight because your liver is refilling with glycogen. As it refills, it pulls in extra fluid. This is normal—it's not fat gain; it is fluid retention! As long as you drink your water and decaffeinated fluid requirement, you will lose the temporary water weight by Day Six. Yes, you will pee a little bit more as your body releases the excess fluid, but you have to drink fluid to lose excess fluid.

Please try putting away your scale and measuring tape for the first eight weeks of Step Two. Follow the program like it's your job: exercise, drink your fluids, get rest, have at least two bags of green tea, and take your supplements. Step Two works! Trust the program.

Instead of having my 11- to 20-gram Carb Dam at meals and bedtime as well as between meals that will exceed five hours, can't I simply eat an 11- to 20-gram Carb Dam every three to four hours? I promise to use my watch!

The right quantity of appropriately timed mild Carb Dams are what Step Two is all about. The rule of Step Two is to use the neutral foods from Step One as your base and then add Carb Dams appropriately.

With that said, you can simply have your 11- to 20-gram Carb Dam every three to four hours, but you might end up with meals that don't get an 11- to 20-gram Carb Dam!

Here's an example of the same day using both methods:

1. Carb Dams at meals, bedtime, and Carb Dams between meals that are more than four to five hours apart.
2. Placing carb dams every three to four hours from wake-up to bedtime.

You can use whatever method appeals to you, as both methods are legal. Personally I like Carb Dams at meals and bedtime plus between meals that are more than four to five hours apart. This way each meal and bedtime has an 11- to 20-gram Carb Dam, and I add an extra 11- to 20-gram carb snack between distant meals to "dam" the liver from releasing glycogen.

I forgot to take an 11- to 20-gram snack when my meals were more than five hours apart. What now?

Every time you go longer than five hours without an 11- to 20-gram Carb Dam your liver releases a meal's worth of glycogen over the next four- to

	Carb Dams at meals, between distant meals, and at bedtime	Carb Dams every four hours
Wake-up	7 a.m.	7 a.m.
Breakfast	7:30 a.m. with 11- to 20-gram Carb Dam	8 a.m. with 11- to 20-gram Dam
Snack	11 a.m. with 11- to 20-gram Carb Dam	12 p.m. with 11- to 20-gram Carb Dam
Lunch	12:45 p.m. with 11- to 20-gram Carb Dam	1:15 p.m. with neutral foods only
Snack	4 p.m. with 11- to 20-gram Carb Dam	4 p.m. with 11- to 20-gram Carb Dam
Dinner	7:30 p.m. with 11- to 20-gram Carb Dam	7 p.m. with neutral foods only
Snack		8 p.m. with 11- to 20-gram Carb Dam
Bedtime snack	11 p.m. with 11- to 20-gram Carb Dam	11 p.m. with 11- to 20-gram Carb Dam
Bedtime	11 p.m.	11 p.m.

five-hour block. This is not one huge dump of glycogen; it is released over the upcoming four to five hours. Your Met B pancreas over-responds to this glycogen dose with excess insulin. So as soon as you realize you missed the five-hour mark, take an 11- to 20-gram Carb Dam. This will dam up the liver and block the four- to five-hour glycogen release. If you realize you've forgotten to take a Carb Dam between distant meals more than three times in a week, you need to return to Step One for a two-week detox to rest your metabolism. Then make a fresh start on Step Two. If you don't rest the overworking pancreas, you will stop losing fat and inches on Step Two.

You are allowed two slip-ups per week after the first two weeks of Step Two have passed. For the first two weeks try for zero slip-ups. From two weeks onward you may choose to have one slip-up per week without needing to revert back to Step One. I teach my patients the Three-Strike Rule: if you've upset the pancreas three or more times (three strikes) in a one-week period, you've "struck out" and need to send your pancreas to a short stint in the "minor leagues" for two weeks in Step One.

Unlike people with Metabolism A who can just restart their diet when they stray off course, those with Metabolism B must start with a clean slate. Return to Step One for two weeks, during which time your pancreas and liver will rest. Then back to Step Two.

I was sick for several days while on Step Two. Although I couldn't eat protein or vegetables, I made sure to eat my 11- to 20-gram Carb Dams. Do I need to do two weeks of Step One to rest the pancreas and liver?

No, you did just the right thing. Remember, MM is a carb-controlled program. We can have protein, fat, and most veggies anytime, but during Step Two our Carb Dams are set up to keep the liver from releasing large amounts of glycogen. You kept your dams up! That's perfect. If you have an unsettled stomach, use easily digested carbs such as 11- to 20-gram net carb crackers, light yogurt, a half banana, or two-third cup of unsweetened natural applesauce, oatmeal, or toast in place of harder-to-digest carbohydrate choices.

Step Two is a more nutritionally balanced way of eating than Step One. Fruit, legumes, whole grains are now part of every day. Should I continue to take my vitamins, minerals, and supplements?

Yes, take them through all three steps of the Metabolism Miracle. Consider your vitamins, minerals, and supplements to be insurance against nutrition deficiencies.

I'm constipated. What do you recommend for Step Two?

Do everything you would do during Step One: drink a minimum of sixty-four ounces of decaffeinated fluid daily, eat raw or al dente vegetables, increase your physical activity, and possibly use a plant fiber supplement. In addition, during Step Two eat fresh fruit with skin intact, and make sure your grain selections contain at least 2 grams of fiber.

I found these incredible oatmeal cookies. Amazingly, each large and chewy cookie has only 16 net carb grams. I'm going to have one cookie as an 11- to 20-gram Carb Dam on Step Two. That's okay, right?

Remember, there's more to choosing an appropriate 11- to 20-gram Carb Dam than finding its net carb grams. On Step Two we make our dense-carb choices based on three points: *net carb grams* between 11 and 20

EVERYTHING YOU SHOULD KNOW ABOUT
PLANT FIBER SUPPLEMENTS

The best way to get fiber into your diet is from natural whole foods. When you eat foods naturally high in dietary fiber (fresh fruit, whole grains with 2 or more grams fiber per serving, legumes, nuts, and fresh veggies), you get the benefit of antioxidants, vitamins, and minerals as well as high fiber.

But some people find it difficult to meet the 25 to 35 grams of fiber per day recommended for healthy fiber intake. If you can't meet the fiber requirement through your daily food intake, you can use a fiber supplement.

Fiber supplements are usually made from plant fiber and come in many forms, including capsules, chewable tablets/wafers (watch for carb grams), and powders. The flavorless powders mix undetected into beverages, yogurt, hot cereal, soup, and even coffee!

Common plant fibers include inulin (not insulin!), oligofructose, psyllium, guar gum, pectin, cellulose, beta-glucan, polydextrose, resistant dextrins, and fructooligosaccharides.

Plant fiber supplements are either soluble or insoluble fiber. Soluble fiber helps lower cholesterol. Insoluble fiber decreases transit time of waste through the GI tract and keeps bowel movements regular.

It is possible to over-do fiber. The result of excess plant fiber is loose stools, diarrhea, bloating, gas, and flatulence. Excess fiber can also bind with necessary minerals and impair their digestion. Although your meal may contain minerals like calcium, iron, and magnesium, excess fiber may stop the absorption of valuable minerals.

To stop your fiber supplement from causing your medications to malabsorb, take the supplement two hours or more after you take your medication.

---

grams, *fiber* over 2 grams, and *sugar* should be less than 6 grams. If your cookie fulfills the three requirements for a Step Two starchy choice, it is just fine. If one of these requirements is absent, the cookie is not the right choice for Step Two.

I keep forgetting to take an 11- to 20-gram Carb Dam between distant meals. Can you suggest anything to help me remember?

Try setting an alarm about four hours after the start of your meal. Some people set an alarm on their computer, iPod, watch, or smartphone. I've even seen patients carry tiny, pocket-sized alarms in their pocket. The alarm will remind you to decide whether you will get your next meal within the allotted five-hour period. If not, you'll know to have an 11- to 20-gram Carb Dam right then and there. Once snacking between distant meals becomes part of your Step Two lifestyle you won't need the alarm. Routinely omitting your necessary between-meal snacks will cause weight gain, backsliding, and a ten-day trip to Step One to clean house.

My best friend wants to try the Metabolism Miracle for weight loss. She has Metabolism A. Is it okay for her to live the MM lifestyle, and will she lose weight?

Although anyone can follow the Metabolism Miracle lifestyle to lose weight, people with Metabolism B get many more rewards that are physical, emotional, and psychological. The Met A person will lose weight (fat) and inches. Remember, the person with Met A does not have insulin imbalance, so they can't expect to feel what a Met B person feels when transitioning from metabolic chaos to normal insulin response. The Metabolism Miracle is one of many weight-reduction plans your friend can follow, but it is the only weight-reduction and health-improvement plan designed especially for those with Met B.

If You Begin to Gain Weight

After every eight-week period of Step Two, you need to reweigh and remeasure. When you check your total weight and inch loss, they should both be within your target range *and* should be within two points of each other. If you lose sixteen pounds and eighteen inches and your target range was fourteen and twenty-one, both your weight and inches are within the target and within two spaces of each other.

But what if, after eight weeks, you only lost ten pounds while your target was fourteen to twenty-one pounds? You have to do a little detective work and find out why your weight and inch loss was lower than expected. There are a handful of reasons that would cause you to lose less pounds and inches than your expected number.

- You've eaten fewer than 11 grams or more than 20 grams of net carb at a meal or snack more than once or twice.
- You've let five hours pass without an 11- to 20-gram Carb Dam.
- You are overly eating proteins and fats.
- You aren't getting a minimum of thirty minutes of exercise five times a week.
- You're suffering from increased stress, a recent illness, or increased pain.
- You've made mistakes on Step Two and did not add necessary slip-up time. If you have more than two slip-ups per week on Step Two, you need to do two weeks of Step One to clean the slate and let your Met B metabolism rest.
- You have hypothyroid (slow metabolism).
- You have chronic high stress.
- You have chronic pain.
- You suffer from an autoimmune or inflammatory disease (rheumatoid arthritis, lupus, Raynaud's syndrome, etc.) and are experiencing a flare-up.

The easiest way to determine why you did not hit your expected weight and inch loss is to keep a detailed two-day food diary that includes the timing of meals and snacks, the foods chosen, and how much of the food you've eaten. You should also note how much and how often you exercise and whether you have suffered any stress, pain, or illness lately.

It's easy to fix forgotten carb servings or to cut down on excessive portions of neutral foods. As for exercise, it's a matter of making up your mind and getting back into your routine. But stress, pain, and sickness are often out of your control and can result in hormonal shifts that cause increases in blood sugar, pancreatic activity, and, ultimately, weight.

You may not be able to control the source of stress, but you may be able to diminish the physical toll it takes on your body. Many people successfully use yoga, deep-breathing techniques, or positive visualization. Others pump up their physical activity to counter increased stress hormones. You can also work with your physician to help minimize chronic pain. One school of thought maintains that waiting too long to treat pain causes additional problems. This line of thinking supports treating pain before it takes its toll on physical and mental health.

Illness triggers the release of stress hormones that are needed for the self-healing process. Unfortunately these hormones cause a natural rise in blood sugar, which causes the pancreas to over-release insulin, the catalyst of weight gain. Take care of yourself with rest, proper nutrition, vitamin and mineral supplementation, decaffeinated fluids, and physical activity to lower your risk of weight regain.

If you realize you have made several errors or were dealing with high stress, illness, or pain while on Step Two, do two weeks of Step One to clean the slate and rest the pancreas and liver. Then weigh, measure, and restart Step Two—without the errors—and see how you fare after eight weeks.

But what if I have chronic conditions, long-term stress, or an autoimmune disease? How will I ever lose weight?

Some people have chronic stressors like autoimmune disease, chronic back pain, frequent migraines, long-term emotional stress, family stress, or inflammatory disease. Consider living in Step One and taking two off-plan meals every month. So you can have pizza or Chinese or Mexican food on your two off-plan meals each month, but instead of reweighing and remeasuring at the end of eight weeks plus time added for slip-ups, you will need to reweigh and remeasure in eight weeks plus twelve days to see whether you have lost within your target range.

There is another way to control the excess glycogen release that will become excess blood glucose when you are stressed emotionally or physically for a long period of time. Ask your physician about using the prescription medication metformin. Metformin has been the number-one prescription medication for type 2 diabetes for many years. (It was previously known as glucophage; metformin is the generic name.)

Metformin does not directly decrease your blood glucose, but it does help decrease the liver's release of glycogen, which helps your pancreas produce less insulin. Metformin is now used for prediabetes (to help prevent the progression to type 2 diabetes) and for PCOS (polycystic ovarian syndrome) to help regulate menstruation and sexual hormone levels. Some physicians are also using metformin for those with metabolic syndrome (Met B) to help improve levels of glucose, blood pressure, cholesterol, triglycerides, and belly fat.

Metformin should always be taken with food. This is a possible schedule for taking metformin; your physician can provide a prescription for you. If you introduce it slowly, you decrease the risk of gas, bloating, diarrhea, and flatulence.

Week one: 500 mg with dinner
Week two: 500 mg with breakfast, 500mg with dinner
Week three: 500 mg with breakfast, 1000mg with dinner.

A typical dose of metformin for PCOS or prediabetes is 1500 mg/day.
A typical dose of metformin for type 2 diabetes is 2000 mg/day.

7

Step Three—
Keeping Fat "Off" and Health "On"
for a Lifetime

Congratulations! After resting and rehabbing your overwrought Metabolism B in Step One and teaching your pancreas and liver to respond normally to a blood glucose rise from carbs and liver release in Step Two, you have reached the weight and clothing size that makes you feel and look great. You have retuned your Metabolism B so it can handle carbohydrates properly, giving your body a healthy future.

As the maintenance step that can easily last a lifetime, Step Three has key benefits, including a wider range of carbohydrate choices. Although the low-impact carb choices from Step Two will *always* be preferable because Step Two carbs, with the exception of milk, yogurt, and fruit, contain over 2 grams of fiber and 6 or fewer grams of sugar, the expanded carb list of Step Three will make occasional treats a possibility, not a slip-up.

One Step at a Time

Here's a recap of the three-step Metabolism Miracle.

Step One: You rested your overworked carbohydrate metabolism by limiting net carbohydrates to the option of a 5-gram Counter Carb at meals, bedtime, and between meals that are more than four to five hours apart. You ate lean protein, heart-healthy fats, and neutral vegetables liberally.

Step Two: You reprogrammed your rested metabolism and delivered yourself to optimal health and your desired weight. You ate a low-impact 11- to 20-gram Carb Dam at intervals of no more than four to five hours. You ate lean protein, heart-healthy fats, and neutral vegetables liberally.

Now with Step Three you will maintain your desired weight, good health, and high energy while adding more choice and flexibility. You will identify the carbohydrate range that works best for your body and choose from an expanded variety of carb choices. You will always consider lean protein, heart-healthy fats, and neutral vegetables to be neutral foods. Always drink adequate water and decaffeinated fluids, take your supplements, drink green tea, exercise, and get adequate rest.

Identifying Your Carb Range

Now that you've reached your desired weight and/or clothing size, you will maintain that weight and size with a carbohydrate range that is specific to your body. In Step Two you limited your net lower-impact carbohydrate choices to 11 to 20 grams at meals, bedtime, and between distant meals so you could continue to lose weight. Step Three is less stringent and allows a more generous daily carb allotment that enables you to maintain your desired weight, size, health, and energy.

To identify a person's ideal carbohydrate range I use a classic nutrition formula that determines the number of calories a person requires

Today marks my two-year anniversary of faithfully following MM. I'm happy to report I have followed the plan, kept the weight off, and I'm still as passionate as ever about living what I call the MM lifestyle. MM has become second nature to me.

I think how much of a lifestyle MM has become to me when I'm taken out of MM context. For example, just recently I was on a business trip and went to the hotel's breakfast buffet. I went about my business, naturally taking some eggs and bringing my own 11-20 gram net carb English muffin. Then I looked around and noticed how much carbohydrate other people were piling up on their plates.

MM has changed me because I made it my life commitment. I follow the plan, always getting back on track if needed. I exercise, drink water, take my vitamins—all things I did not do before.

I have also made substitutions for favorite foods, but that does not bother me at all because on MM I lost my carb cravings. My labs also tell the real story of what is going on because of my dedication to MM: at fifty-one, I'm no longer on any medications!

—*Lynne*

to maintain their desired weight, neither gaining nor losing. Because a person with Metabolism B does not maintain weight solely by counting calories, I modified the classic formula to match the requirements of Metabolism B. When all the calculating is through, a person with Metabolism B will consume from 30 to 35 percent of their calories from carbohydrate foods and, in the spirit of a balanced diet, 30 to 35 percent from protein and fat too.

You can quickly find your *maximum* number of daily carb servings to maintain your desired weight by pinpointing your sex, height, age, desired maintenance weight, and activity level in the following tables (pages 148–150). This is a very individualized way to determine carbs rather than a one-size-fits-all chart. This easy method will allow both a six-foot-six, eighteen-year-old high school basketball player and his five-foot-one, sedentary, seventy-year-old grandma to figure out the right amount of net carb for each of them.

The key to Step Three is to spread your carb servings throughout the day appropriately. You'll still think in terms of five-hour intervals because that's how the liver works. And you'll have to be careful to get enough but not too many carb servings in any of those five-hour intervals. Eating too few carbs at a meal or snack allows the liver to kick in and release its glycogen stores. But eating too many carbs at a meal or snack will cause the rested pancreas to overreact. Both create havoc with Metabolism B and ultimately lead to weight gain.

To prevent such hiccups in Step Three, remember these simple rules.

Three Simple Rules for Step Three

1. One carb serving is the *minimum* you may take at a meal, bedtime, or required snack.
2. Four carb servings are the *maximum* you may take at a meal, bedtime, or required snack.

CARB CHARTS

FEMALE
Height: 5'0" to 5'3"
Maintenance weight: 100 to 130 pounds

Age	Activity	Maximum Carb Servings per Day
teens to 20	low	8.5
	moderate	9
	high	9.5
20s and 30s	low	8
	moderate	8.5
	high	9
40s and 50s	low	7.5
	moderate	8
	high	8.5
60s and 70s	low	7
	moderate	7.5
	high	8
over 80	low	6.5
	moderate	7
	high	7.5

FEMALE
Height: 5'4" to 5'7"
Maintenance weight: 120 to 150 pounds

Age	Activity	Maximum Carb Servings per Day
teens to 20	low	9.5
	moderate	10
	high	10.5
20s and 30s	low	9
	moderate	9.5
	high	10
40s and 50s	low	8.5
	moderate	9
	high	9.5
60s and 70s	low	8
	moderate	8.5
	high	9
over 80	low	7.5
	moderate	8
	high	8.5

FEMALE
Height: 5'8" to 5'11"
Maintenance weight: 140 to 170 pounds

Age	Activity	Maximum Carb Servings per Day
teens to 20	low	10
	moderate	11
	high	12
20s and 30s	low	9.5
	moderate	10.5
	high	11.5
40s and 50s	low	9
	moderate	10
	high	11
60s and 70s	low	8.5
	moderate	9.5
	high	10.5
over 80	low	8
	moderate	9
	high	10

FEMALE
Height: 6'0" to 6'3"
Maintenance weight: 155 to 185 pounds

Age	Activity	Maximum Carb Servings per Day
teens to 20	low	11
	moderate	12
	high	13
20s and 30s	low	10.5
	moderate	11.5
	high	12.5
40s and 50s	low	10
	moderate	11
	high	12
60s and 70s	low	9.5
	moderate	10.5
	high	11.5
over 80	low	9
	moderate	10
	high	11

CARB CHARTS

MALE
Height: 5'0" to 5'3"
Maintenance weight: 106 to 136 pounds

Age	Activity	Maximum Carb Servings per Day
teens to 20	low	9
	moderate	10
	high	11
20s and 30s	low	8.5
	moderate	9.5
	high	10.5
40s and 50s	low	8
	moderate	9
	high	10
60s and 70s	low	7.5
	moderate	8.5
	high	9.5
over 80	low	7
	moderate	8
	high	9

MALE
Height: 5'4" to 5'7"
Maintenance weight: 130 to 160 pounds

Age	Activity	Maximum Carb Servings per Day
teens to 20	low	10
	moderate	11
	high	12
20s and 30s	low	9.5
	moderate	10.5
	high	11.5
40s and 50s	low	9
	moderate	10
	high	11
60s and 70s	low	8.5
	moderate	9.5
	high	10.5
over 80	low	8
	moderate	9
	high	10

MALE
Height: 5'8" to 5'11"
Maintenance weight: 154 to 185 pounds

Age	Activity	Maximum Carb Servings per Day
teens to 20	low	11
	moderate	12
	high	13
20s and 30s	low	10.5
	moderate	11.5
	high	12.5
40s and 50s	low	10
	moderate	11
	high	12
60s and 70s	low	9.5
	moderate	10.5
	high	11.5
over 80	low	9
	moderate	10
	high	11

MALE
Height: 6'0" to 6'3"
Maintenance weight: 178 to 210 pounds

Age	Activity	Maximum Carb Servings per Day
teens to 20	low	12
	moderate	13
	high	14
20s and 30s	low	11.5
	moderate	12.5
	high	13.5
40s and 50s	low	11
	moderate	12
	high	13
60s and 70s	low	10.5
	moderate	11.5
	high	12.5
over 80	low	10
	moderate	11
	high	12

CARB CHARTS

MALE		
Height: 6'3" to 6'6"		
Maintenance weight: 196 to 235 pounds		
Age	Activity	Maximum Carb Servings per Day
teens to 20	low	13
	moderate	14
	high	15
20s and 30s	low	12.5
	moderate	13.5
	high	14.5
40s and 50s	low	12
	moderate	13
	high	14
60s and 70s	low	11.5
	moderate	12.5
	high	13.5
over 80	low	11
	moderate	12
	high	13

MALE		
Height: over 6'6"		
Maintenance weight: 226 to 250 pounds		
Age	Activity	Maximum Carb Servings per Day
teens to 20	low	14
	moderate	15
	high	16
20s and 30s	low	13.5
	moderate	14.5
	high	15.5
40s and 50s	low	13
	moderate	14
	high	15
60s and 70s	low	12.5
	moderate	13.5
	high	14.5
over 80	low	12
	moderate	12
	high	14

3. Your total carb servings in a day should not exceed your personal maximum carb servings but can be fewer than your maximum as long as all of your carb needs are met.

Let's follow Lisa, the forty-nine-year-old mother with a maintenance amount of carbs of nine servings per day. In her work as a local TV personality, she is often rushed in the morning, has a quick lunch at her desk, has an afternoon snack on the way home, usually makes dinner at home, and exercises after dinner. During the work week she distributes her maximum nine carb servings something like this:

6:30 a.m.: Wake up
7:00 a.m.: Breakfast—2 carb servings
12:00 p.m.: Lunch—2 carb servings
4:00 p.m.: Midafternoon snack—1 carb serving
7:00 p.m.: Dinner—2 or 3 carb servings

ONE SIZE DOES NOT FIT ALL IN THE FAMILY

Even if all members of your family have Metabolism B, everyone's Step Three will have a different number of carb servings per day. The number will be based on gender, age, height, desired weight, and activity.

Dad: At age fifty and standing at six feet tall, Phil has reached his desired weight of 206 pounds using the first two Steps of MM. He now runs or bikes five mornings a week for fifty minutes to one hour before heading off to work. On the Carb Chart a man of Phil's age, height, and moderate activity level needs a *maximum of 12 carb servings a day* to maintain his 206 pounds.

Mom: Lisa, forty-nine years old and five-foot-five, has type 2 diabetes but has her blood glucose under control since finishing eight weeks on Step One of the Metabolism Miracle. She feels great at 143 pounds, and she reached that weight at the end of Step Two. Lisa takes a brisk walk every evening for forty-five minutes to an hour and takes the occasional bike ride on the weekend and walk with her daughter. On the Carb Chart a woman of Lisa's age, height, and moderate activity level can use up to *9 carb servings a day* to maintain her weight.

Daughter: As an undergraduate college student, twenty-one-year-old Diana is five-foot-four and has maintained her desired weight of 130 pounds for several years.

Four nights per week Diana does a hard workout at a nearby fitness center that lasts over an hour. On weekends she takes a walk with her mom. With her high activity level, Diana can eat up to *10 carb servings per day* without gaining weight. During exam week, when she can't find the time to get to the gym and her activity level enters the low zone, Diana limits her carbs to 9 servings per day.

Son: Eighteen-year-old Phillip is a starter on his varsity high school football team. Between practice and the games, he works out six days a week for more than two hours each time. According to the Carb Chart, at six-foot-one and 220 pounds, a muscular teenager with Phillip's high activity level can eat up to 14 carb servings a day without gaining weight. As he desires to maintain a slightly higher weight (muscle mass) during football season, he then adds 1 carb serving to the 14 he is allotted for his height, weight, and activity level, consuming 15 carb servings per day. During the off-season Phillip still works out five days a week for at least forty-five minutes, but at this moderate activity level he decreases his carb servings to 13 per day.

8:15 p.m.: Exercise
10:30 p.m.: Bedtime snack—1 carb serving
11:15 p.m.: Sleep
Total carb servings: 8 or 9

Following Steps Three's basic rules, Lisa keeps her carb servings at meals and snacks to at least one and not more than four. When meals are more than five hours apart, her between-meal snack has at least one carb serving.

On the weekend Lisa's schedule is quite different. She eats a pre-exercise snack in the early morning, enjoys a leisurely breakfast when she's done with her bike ride, has a light lunch, afternoon snack, goes out for dinner, and then munches on a light snack before bed. Her carb placement for the weekend follows this schedule:

6:45 a.m.: Wake up
7:00 a.m.: Pre-exercise snack—1 carb serving
7:45 a.m.: Bike ride
9:30 a.m.: Breakfast—2 carb servings
1:30 p.m.: Lunch—1 carb serving
4:30 p.m.: Midafternoon snack—1 carb serving
8:00 p.m.: Dinner—3 carb servings
12:00 a.m.: Bedtime snack—1 carb serving
Total carb servings: 9

On a recent Monday Lisa felt under the weather and spent the day resting at home. She kept to the rule of at least one carb serving at every meal, bedtime, and snacks as needed, but she had no desire to eat her maximum nine carb servings. Instead, she ate one carb serving at all meals and snacks except dinner, when she ate two.

8:30 a.m.: Wake up
9:00 a.m.: Breakfast—1 carb serving
1:00 p.m.: Lunch—1 carb serving
4:30 p.m.: Midafternoon snack—1 carb serving
7:00 p.m.: Dinner—2 carb serving
10:00 p.m.: Bedtime snack—1 carb serving
Total carb servings: 6

Lisa's daughter, Diana, who consumes a maximum of ten carb servings a day, has developed an eating schedule for the school week. On her typical school day:

9:00 a.m.: Wake up
9:45 a.m.: Snack and off to class—1 carb serving
2:30 p.m.: Lunch—2 carb servings
5:00 p.m.: Snack—2 carb servings
6:00 p.m.: Exercise
7:30 p.m.: Dinner—3 to 4 carb servings
12 a.m.: Snack—1 carb serving
Total carb servings: 9 to 10

Because of her upcoming spring break, Diana takes her carb allotment to a lower range for bikini season:

7:00 a.m.: Wake up
7:30 a.m.: Breakfast—1 carb serving
12:00 p.m.: Lunch—1 carb serving
4:00 p.m.: Midafternoon snack—1 carb serving
7:00 p.m.: Dinner—2 carb servings
11:00 p.m.: Bedtime snack—1 carb serving
Total carb servings: 6

In both cases Diana follows the basic rules, with no meal or snack containing less than one carb serving or more than four servings, and she has not exceeded her ten carb servings per day.

Two Types of Carb Servings in Step Three:
Low or High Impact!

Now that you know the maximum number of carb servings that will maintain your ideal weight, take a look at the Step Three carbohydrates list (page 155). Carb choices from Step Two remain on the list, but there are expanded choices and two types of carbohydrate foods in each category: *low impact* and *high impact*. I still recommend the low-impact

WHAT IS A CARB "SERVING"?

One carb serving is the amount of any food with 11 to 20 grams net carb. To make it easy, you can think of one carb serving as containing an average of 15 grams net carb.

In Step One, to rest your pancreas and liver, you had the option of having a 5-gram Counter Carb at meals, bedtime, and between distant meals.

In Step Two, to keep your pancreas from over-releasing insulin and your liver from releasing glycogen stores, you were required to have a Carb Dam (11 to 20 net grams of low-impact carb) at each meal, bedtime, and when time between meals exceeded five hours.

In Step Three you have the most flexibility. Simply find your maximum number of carb servings per day, and *you* choose to distribute them the way you want for the day with a few simple rules.

The basic rule for spacing your carbohydrate servings on Step Three is that you should have at least one carb serving at a meal, bedtime, or required snack when time between meals exceeds five hours, but don't consume more than four servings at one meal, bedtime, or required snack: "minimum of one serving, maximum of four servings"—if your carb servings permit. You needn't use your maximum number of carb servings every day, but you can hit your maximum every day if you want to.

Most people enjoy thinking in terms of carb servings, knowing that each carb serving contains 11 to 20 grams net carb (with an average of 15 grams net carb). So four carb servings is equivalent to 60 grams of carb (4 x 15 = 60), and three carb servings is equivalent to 45 grams of carb (3 x 15 = 45). If you know the number of net carb grams in an item, divide by 15 to find the carb servings it contains. So 60 grams net carb divided by 15 equals four carb servings.

choices (2 or more grams of fiber and 6 or fewer grams of sugar per serving), but on Step Three you may *occasionally* choose a high-impact food. These are not the most nutritious choices, and their higher glycemic index or lower fiber grams will cause your pancreas to stir more than low-impact carbs do.

Step Three Carbohydrates

All portions are one carb serving, or 11 to 20 grams net carb.

Breads
Low Impact (2 or more grams of fiber and 6 or fewer grams of sugar)

2 slices of light, thin-sliced whole-grain bread

1 slice of whole-grain bread

1 light whole-grain English muffin

½ whole-grain English muffin

1 light or low-carb whole-grain pita

½ whole-grain pita

High Impact

One 1-ounce slice of white, whole-wheat, rye, or pumpernickel bread

1 ounce of bakery bread, rolls, buns, and so forth

1 hot dog roll

½ burger bun

½ pita

¾ ounce of matzo

One 1-ounce chapatti or roti (use food scale)

One 1-ounce mini-bagel or mini-muffin

1 fajita shell

1 soft taco shell

2 hard taco shells

1 frozen waffle

Two 4-inch pancakes

Breading

One 2-inch cube of corn bread

1 ounce of bakery bread (use a food scale)

¾ cup of croutons

Cereals and Grains
Low Impact (2 or more grams of fiber and 6 or fewer grams of sugar)

½ cup of cooked oatmeal

½ cup of cooked barley

BIG BAGEL BONANZA

Big isn't always better. A tiny mini-bagel contains one carb serving, but the standard four-ounce bagel most Americans eat packs four carb servings! Place a bagel, bakery bread, or rolls on a food scale—every ounce it weighs is one carb serving. When I have a bagel or bakery buns or rolls, I always scoop out the middle. A four-ounce bagel can become a two-ounce bagel by removing the inside.

Don't forget to count the breading on fish or chicken too. The breading on most items counts as one carb serving.

½ cup of cooked brown or wild rice
½ cup of cooked whole-grain pasta (cooked al dente)
½ cup of cooked bulgur
1 serving of dry cereal (check the Nutrition Label to make sure it is a
   low-impact carb)

High Impact
   ½ cup of cooked cream of wheat
   ½ cup of cooked farina
   ½ cup of cooked quinoa
   ½ cup of cooked grits
   ⅓ cup of cooked white rice
   ½ cup of basmati rice
   ⅓ cup of cooked white pasta
   ½ cup of pasta salad
   ½ cup of macaroni and cheese
   ½ cup of casserole dish made with pasta

Crackers and Starchy Snacks
Low Impact (2 or more grams of fiber and 6 or fewer grams of sugar)
   1 serving of whole-grain crackers
   3 cups of popcorn (light or hot air–popped, with no partially
      hydrogenated oils or trans fats)

1 serving of whole-grain pretzels

1 serving of tortilla chips

1 serving of whole-grain pretzels

High Impact

1 serving of any kind of crackers with 11 to 20 grams net carb

1 serving of chips with 11 to 20 grams net carb

1 serving of pretzels with 11 to 20 grams net carb

1½ oblong graham crackers (3 squares)

4 slices of melba toast

2 large rice cakes

8 small rice cakes

6 saltines

½ cup of chow mein noodles

3 sandwich crackers with cheese or peanut butter filling

Countable Vegetables and Legumes

Low Impact

½ cup of corn

½ ear of fresh corn

½ cup of peas

½ cup of legumes such as kidney beans, lentils, lima beans, chickpeas, white beans, black beans, or white kidney beans

½ cup of hummus

1½ cups of carrots

½ sweet potato or yam or ½ cup of mashed sweet potato or yam

1½ cups of cooked carrots or 1½ cups of raw carrots

1 cup of beets

1 cup of rutabaga

High Impact

½ cup of mashed potatoes

½ baked white potato

3 ounces of boiled potato

½ small order of French fries

½ cup of potato salad

½ cup of baked beans

¼ cup of mashed plantain

1 cup of winter or acorn squash

Soups

Low Impact

1 cup of tomato soup (water-based)

½ cup of lentil soup

½ cup of split-pea soup

1 cup of greens and beans

1 cup of chili with beans

1 cup of chicken noodle soup with whole-grain noodles or brown rice

1 cup of cream soup—spinach, broccoli, chicken, onion with no potatoes (high fat)

High Impact

1 cup of broth-based soup with noodles, potatoes, rice, or barley

1 cup of cream soup with potatoes (high in fat)

½ cup of pasta e fagioli soup

½ cup of minestrone soup

Protein Bars

Low Impact

A protein bar is a low-impact carb if it contains 11 to 20 grams net carb and has 2 or more grams fiber and 6 or fewer grams of sugar.

High Impact

A protein bar is a high-impact carb if it contains 11 to 20 grams net carb. Many protein bars have more than 6 grams added sugar.

Fruit

All portions represent 11 to 20 grams net carb. Fruit choices should be average in size. You can also just count a serving of fruit as 15 grams net carb.

Low Impact

1 apple (medium, 3-inch diameter)

4 dried apple rings

1 pear (small or ½ large pear)

1 peach (medium or 3-inch diameter)

2 plums (medium or 2 ⅛ -inch diameter)

1 nectarine (medium or 3-inch diameter)

15 medium or 12 large cherries

⅔ cup natural applesauce (read the Nutrition Facts label for total carb minus fiber—don't look at sugar)

½ grapefruit (4- to 5-inch diameter for full fruit; AVOID if you are taking the statin Lipitor)

1 cup of sliced strawberries

1 cup of blackberries

1 cup of blueberries

1 cup of raspberries

2 clementine oranges or 2 small tangerines

4 apricots or 8 dried apricot halves

15 medium or 12 large grapes

1 orange

1 cup (4 ounces) of pineapple cubes

½ medium banana

High Impact

  3 dates

  2 figs

  1 kiwi

  ½ small mango

  ½ cup of cubed mango

  1 cup of cubed papaya or ½ papaya

  3 prunes

  40 raisins

  dried fruit (11 to 20 grams net carb)

  1 cup of honeydew melon balls or cubes

  1 cup of cantaloupe melon balls or cubes (about ⅓ cantaloupe)

  1½ cups of watermelon balls or cubes

  1 cup of guava

Milk and Other Dairy

All portions represent 11 to 20 grams net carb.

Low Impact

    1 cup (8 fluid ounces) of fat-free, nonfat, 1%, 2%, or skim-plus milk

    1 carb serving of plain yogurt

    ½ cup of sugar-free, fat-free pudding

    1 carb serving of fruit-flavored yogurt sweetened with sucralose, stevia, or Splenda

    1 carb serving of no-sugar-added ice cream sweetened with Splenda

High Impact

    ½ cup of ice cream (light, low-fat, or regular)

    ½ cup of frozen yogurt (light or regular)

Occasional Treats

These high-impact carbs are loaded with fat and have little nutritional benefit. Still, they can be a tasty treat from time to time. Each is shown in a typical serving size with its carb servings listed beside it.

    1 brownie, unfrosted (4-inch square): 2 carb servings

    1 brownie, frosted (4-inch square): 4 carb servings

    Cake, unfrosted (4-inch square): 2 carb servings

    Cake, frosted (4-inch square): 4 carb servings

    2 sandwich-type cookies with filling in the middle: 1 carb serving

    2 cookies, average size, homemade, such as chocolate chip: 1 carb serving

    1 frosted cupcake (small): 2 carb servings

    1 plain cake doughnut: 2 carb servings

    1 glazed-type doughnut: 2 carb servings

    ⅛ double-crusted fruit pie: 3 carb servings

    ⅛ single-crusted fruit pie: 2 carb servings

    ⅛ pumpkin or custard pie: 2 carb servings

    ⅛ large pizza: 3 carb servings

    ⅛ large pizza, thick outer edge of crust removed: 2 carb servings

    1 bagel: 4 carb servings

    ½ bagel: 2 carb servings

    1 hollowed-out bagel: 2 carb servings

    1 hard roll, Kaiser roll, or 6-inch sub roll: 3 carb servings

    1 hollowed-out hard roll, Kaiser roll, or sub roll: 2 carb servings

1 wrap: 3 carb servings

1 cup of a casserole dish such as lasagna, macaroni and cheese, tuna
   casserole: 2 carb servings

Small order of fries: 2 carb servings

Medium order of fries: 3 carb servings

Large order of fries: 4 carb servings

1 breaded fish sandwich on a bun: 3 carb servings

1 breaded chicken sandwich on a bun: 3 carb servings

1 bun for large burgers or fast-food sandwiches: 3 carb servings

6 chicken nuggets: 1 carb serving

6 pieces of sushi: 1 carb serving

1 cup of Chinese food such as beef and broccoli, shrimp and veggies
   with sauce, but no rice or noodles: 1 carb serving

1 cup of Chinese rice, white or fried: 3 carb servings

Sauce or gravy: 1 carb serving

2 wontons: 1 carb serving

Breading on any food: 1 carb serving

A Day in the Life of Step Three

Let's see how several more people handle the Step Three distribution of
their daily carbs.

Mike's Step Three

Mike is a thirty-three-year-old policeman. When he joined the police department ten years ago he was a strapping five-foot-eleven, 165-pound,
twenty-three-year-old guy who could get away with eating anything he
liked. Time caught up with Mike. Eight years into his career he was a
thirty-one-year-old man with a wife, two kids, a mortgage, and lots of
stress. His physical activity had decreased to nothing, he was up to 194
pounds, and his eating habits were out of control. As a policeman, he
joked that "it's true what they say about donuts and cops." But inside
Mike was very unhappy with his body.

He began following the Metabolism Miracle after his thirty-first birthday and made a habit of spending thirty to forty-five minutes in the gym
five days a week. After two rounds of Step Two he had gotten down to 171

CHANGING NET CARB GRAMS INTO THE
NUMBER OF CARB SERVINGS

When you are food shopping you may find a packaged product with Nutrition Facts and feel uncertain whether you can fit it into Step Three of your program. Keep in mind that foods with fiber of two or more grams and sugar of 6 or fewer grams per serving are always the *best* choices for a person with Met B.

Here's how to turn a product's net carb grams into carb servings for Step Three. From the Nutrition Facts label:

1. Check serving size.
2. Total carb grams minus dietary fiber grams equals net carb grams.
3. Now, simply divide the net carb grams by 15 to find your carb servings.

For example:

Frozen Pizza
Serving size = 1 slice (1/8 of the pizza pie)
Total carbohydrate: 48 grams
Dietary fiber: 2 grams
48 grams carb – 2 grams fiber = 46 grams net carb
46 ÷ 15 = 3 carb servings

One slice of this frozen pizza has three carb servings.

pounds and could no longer fit into his uniform, no matter how tightly he pulled his belt. According to the Carb Chart, Mike's allotment for his weight maintenance is 10.5 carb servings per day. Here's how he spreads out those servings.

5:45 a.m.: Wake up
6:00 a.m.: Breakfast—2 carb servings: hollowed-out bagel (2 carb servings) with light cream cheese; coffee with half-and-half and Splenda
9:30 a.m.: Midmorning snack—1 carb serving: 1 peach (1 carb serving) with a handful of nuts

Large Bran Muffin
Serving size = ½ muffin
Total carbohydrate: 32 grams
Dietary fiber: 2 grams
Sugar: 5 grams
32 grams carb – 2 grams fiber = 30 grams net carb
30 ÷ 15 = 2 carb servings

So half of the bran muffin contains two carb servings and is a mild-impact carb, as it has 2 grams of fiber and 5 grams of sugar. But if you eat the whole muffin, you are using four carb servings and consuming 10 grams of sugar!

Rice pudding
Serving size = 1 container (½ cup)
Total carbohydrate: 24 grams
Dietary fiber: 1 gram
Sugar: 8 grams
24 grams carb – 1 gram fiber = 23 grams net carb
23 ÷ 15 = 1½ carb servings

So half of a cup of rice pudding contains 1.5 carb servings, though it's a high-impact carb, as it has over 6 grams of sugar and fewer than 2 grams of fiber. You may have it on Step Three, but don't overdo it!

12:30 p.m.: Lunch—2 carb servings: 2 slices of whole-wheat bread (2 carb servings) with sliced turkey breast, Swiss cheese, lettuce and tomato, and "light on the mayo"

4:40 p.m.: Midafternoon snack—½ carb serving: 6 cherries (½ carb serving); handful of peanuts

6:00 p.m.: Dinner—4 carb servings: garden salad with light ranch dressing; grilled chicken; 1 baked potato (2 carb servings) with whipped butter and light sour cream; 1 ear of corn (2 carb servings)

10:00 p.m.: Bedtime snack—1 carb serving: 1 light multigrain English muffin (1 carb serving) spread with natural peanut butter

If you'd rather avoid doing the math to determine carb servings from carb grams, tuck this cheat sheet into your wallet or handbag for easy reference. Once you know the net grams of a food you can find that number on this chart, and the conversion of net carb grams to carb servings is done for you.

If your net carbs are . . . , then your carb servings are . . .

5.5 to 10 grams = ½ carb serving

11 to 20 grams = 1 carb serving

21 to 25 grams = 1½ carb servings

26 to 35 grams = 2 carb servings

36 to 40 grams = 2½ carb servings

41 to 50 grams = 3 carb servings

51 to 55 grams = 3½ carb servings

56 to 65 grams = 4 carb servings

More than 65 grams of carb = TOO MUCH!

Barbara's Step Three

Barbara is a seventy-year-old grandmother of three. At her annual physical exam she was five-foot-three and weighed 166 pounds. Her physician mentioned that if she lost 7 percent of her body weight (about eleven to twelve pounds), she might be able to reduce or even eliminate her medications for hypertension and cholesterol.

Barb started the Metabolism Miracle program and signed up for her community's walking club. She and her friends walked after breakfast for thirty to forty minutes, four to five mornings per week.

After Step Two Barb weighed 145 pounds. She looked as if she weighed 135 pounds and was thrilled with the way she looked and felt. Best of all, with her 18-pound fat loss, her physician was able to discontinue her medications. According to the Carb Chart, Barb's allotment is seven carb servings for weight maintenance.

Here's how Barb chose to spread her seven carb servings.

6:45 a.m.: Wake up

7:00 a.m.: Breakfast—1 carb serving: 2 slices of thin-sliced whole-wheat toast (1 carb serving) with whipped butter; egg white omelet; herbal tea with stevia

8:30 a.m.: Exercise: walking about thirty to forty minutes, 16 ounces of water

9:30 a.m.: Midmorning snack—1 carb serving: 1 peach (1 carb serving); handful of almonds

1:00 p.m.: Lunch—1 carb serving: 1 low-carb wrap (5 grams net carb) filled with tuna salad made with light mayonnaise plus lettuce and sliced tomato; 1 apple (1 carb serving; 5 grams from wrap plus 15 grams from apple = 1 carb serving); diet soda with Splenda

4:30 p.m.: Midafternoon snack—1 carb serving: 1 serving of light yogurt (1 carb serving); lemon infused water

7:00 p.m.: Dinner, dining out—2 carb servings: 5 ounces of wine (with MD's okay); grilled flounder; large garden salad with balsamic vinaigrette; broccoli spears; baked potato (2 carb servings) with whipped butter or light sour cream

11:00 p.m.: Bedtime snack—1 carb serving: 1 cup of blueberries with light whipped cream (1 carb serving)

Barb used all of her seven carb servings for the day!

If You Begin to Gain Weight

The ease and flexibility of Step Three allows you to vary your carb intake within your maximum range and have tremendous freedom with your carb choices. Meanwhile lean protein, heart-healthy fats, and neutral vegetables continue to be neutral. Maintaining your weight is an indication that you are eating a very reasonable amount of protein, fat, and veggies and getting adequate physical activity.

If, despite staying within the limitations of your maximum carb servings per day, your weight begins to creep up, you need to take a moment to analyze the situation. There are only a handful of reasons that would cause your weight to increase:

- You regularly exceeded your maximum carb servings per day.

- You've eaten fewer than 11 grams of net carb at a meal or snack on more than one occasion.
- You've let more than five hours pass without having at least one carb serving.
- You are overeating proteins and fats (especially pay attention to limiting excess fat).
- You aren't getting thirty minutes of exercise five times a week.
- You're suffering from increased stress, a recent illness, or increased pain.
- You have a slow thyroid (hypothyroidism).
- You may require a prescription for metformin.

The easiest way to determine why your weight might be creeping up is to keep a detailed two-day food diary that includes the timing of meals and snacks, the foods chosen, and how much of the food you've eaten. You should also note how much and how often you exercise and whether you have suffered any stress, pain, or illness lately.

When you review your two-day food diary, ask yourself:

____ Are the portion sizes of carbohydrate choices correct?

____ Are there gaps of over five hours without a carb serving?

____ Did I forget to take a carb serving within an hour of waking up?

____ Did I skip a carb serving within one hour of bedtime?

____ Am I overeating neutral foods?

____ Did I exercise adequately?

____ Am I unusually stressed?

____ Am I in pain?

____ Am I feeling ill?

____ Do I suffer from autoimmune or inflammatory disease (rheumatoid arthritis, lupus, Raynaud's syndrome, etc.) and am I experiencing a flare-up?

____ Do I have hypothyroidism?

It's easy to fix forgotten carb servings or to cut down on excessive portions of neutral foods. As for exercise, it's a matter of making up your mind and getting back into your routine. But stress, pain, and sickness are often out of your control and can result in hormonal shifts that cause increases in blood sugar, pancreatic activity, and, ultimately, weight.

Another way to control weight is to decrease excess glycogen release due to long-term stress, pain, or illness; see page 117 in Step Two for ways to counteract these. You can ask your MD about a prescription for the drug metformin. (For more about metformin, see pages 142–143.)

A Quick Mention of Slip-Ups

You're bound to have a few slip-ups as you live the MM lifestyle. If you come back from vacation, after the holidays, a harried time in your life, illness, high stress, a flare-up of an autoimmune disease, time on steroids, or pain, remember to reset your metabolism with two weeks of Step One followed by two weeks of Step Two before returning to Step Three.

Step Three: Frequently Asked Questions

Steps One and Two are weight- and fat-loss Steps. What does Step Three achieve?

When you have reached your own personal desired weight and size, feel great, like the way you look, and take as little medication as possible, Step Three will maintain this for a lifetime. It allows an expanded range of carb types and gives you the flexibility to place carb servings where you want as long as you have a minimum of one serving (and a max of four servings) at meals and necessary snacks.

Even if I am allowed a maximum of ten carb servings per day, should I stick closer to eight servings a day?

Any carbohydrate amount within your maintenance range is perfectly fine. You needn't deprive yourself by staying to one carb serving per meal when you desire two or three. Just be sure you don't regularly exceed your maximum carb servings per day.

My jeans are getting snug in the waist. What's the quickest way to return to my comfortable, healthy size?

Weight gain for people with Metabolism B is not usually a function of excess calories but rather of excess insulin and inadequate exercise. Create a two-day food diary and identify what might be causing the fat gain. Once you have found the culprit, you will need to detox, with two weeks on Step One to rest your metabolism followed by two weeks on Step Two to reprogram it.

Now that I'm on the maintenance portion of my plan for life, should I continue taking supplements and drinking green tea?

I wish I could tell you that you can get all of your needed vitamins, minerals, and antioxidants from the foods you eat. It is my opinion that our food supply is overprocessed and tinkered with chemically and hormonally. It's more than probable that we can easily miss out on some of the vitamins and minerals we need. I think of MM's supplements and recommendation for green tea as insurance that your body gets what it needs.

Can I ever ease back into a "normal" lifestyle, or will I be forever timing my meals, counting carbs, and reading food labels?

The Metabolism Miracle is the "normal" way of life for anyone with Metabolism B. If you eat haphazardly, your pancreas will overreact with excess insulin, you will regain weight, and you will begin to experience all the symptoms that fluctuating blood sugar once caused: fatigue, depression, anxiety, restless sleep, midline fat, blurry vision, irritability, and carb cravings. In time you could develop type 2 diabetes and require daily medications for many weight-related medical conditions.

Don't think of the Metabolism Miracle as a quick fix or just another weight-loss program; it is the healthiest lifestyle for a person born with your metabolism. It will keep you at your healthy weight and size on the least amount of medication.

I have two children who seem to be manifesting Metabolism B. My daughter is nine and my son is thirteen. Is it wise for them to begin the program now?

Growing children require a balanced diet for proper growth and their increased energy demands. I'm reluctant to start young children on the Metabolism Miracle program because Step One is not a balanced diet. I rarely recommend the program to boys until they have reached the age of eighteen, when much of their growth is complete, or for girls until at least two years after their first menstrual period.

If their pediatrician orders a blood panel that includes a metabolic panel, thyroid panel, lipid panel, and HbA1C and finds that their numbers point to Metabolism B, I would not hesitate to put a child on four weeks of Step One followed by Step Two until healthy weight and labs are attained. They can follow the rules of Step Three for life with no problem whatsoever.

Your child's pediatrician should help with determining healthy weight, and a registered dietitian can figure out a healthy carb allotment (30 to 35 percent) using a pediatric calorie formula.

If their labs are normal and they are too young to begin the entire Metabolism Miracle program, you can still teach them healthy eating patterns:

- Start each day with breakfast that includes lean protein and is not excessive in carbohydrate content. Think scrambled eggs with half the yolks removed, a light multigrain English muffin, half of a banana, and a glass of unsweetened almond milk.
- Encourage healthy lower-carb snacks between meals, such as natural peanut butter, low-fat cheese sticks, low-carb yogurt, or lean turkey roll-ups.
- Get them into the habit of having a healthy snack before bed that includes lean protein and perhaps a high-fiber starch such as peanut butter on whole-wheat toast and a glass of milk or light yogurt and whole-grain crackers with 11 to 20 grams net carb.
- Limit high-impact carb snacks, including white-flour products, crackers, potato chips, white-flour pretzels, cookies, and candy.
- Eliminate fruit juice and soda from your home. Let your children get their fruit requirement from a piece of fresh fruit instead, and get into the habit of drinking water.
- Avoid giving children and teenagers artificial sweeteners or caffeine. Consider using half the sugar in a recipe.

- I recommend parents shop for carbs recommended in the Step Two lists. These are the highest in nutrition and fiber and lowest in sugar!

In Step Two I get my base of protein, healthy fat, neutral veggies and an 11- to 20-gram net carb serving at all my meals, bedtime, and snacks. I usually consume 6 to 7 carb servings a day on Step Two, and Step Three's Carb Chart recommends a maximum of 9.5 carb servings a day for my age and activity level. I'm worried about regaining weight and want to stay in Step Two!

Step Two is a weight- and fat-loss step. If you continue to follow Step Two's guidelines, you will continue to lose weight. If you are at your desired weight, like the way you look and feel, and your labs and blood pressure are normal when you are on as little medication as possible, you should become familiar with your maintenance plan. How about giving yourself a little leeway and indulge in your full complement of maintenance carb servings once or twice a week?

I easily maintain my carb grams according to Step Three's few rules, but I would REALLY like to know how many ounces of lean protein and how many servings of fat I should have in a day. Doesn't it make a difference?

There is no reason for you to weigh protein and measure fat servings if you are following any step of MM. If you find that you are gaining weight and you are certain your carb intake is correct, start by increasing your exercise or changing the type of exercise *and* decreasing your added fat intake (including salad dressing, oil, mayonnaise, nuts, nut butter, olives, avocado, butter, sour cream, cream cheese, etc.). Fat is very calorie dense. One teaspoon of butter (one pat) has fifty calories! Your body will burn the excess fat in your daily intake before it burns fat from your body.

What about the holidays? Is there an MM holiday plan so I can join in the holiday celebrations without gaining weight? I've been known to gain eight to ten pounds between Thanksgiving and New Years Day!

THE MM PLAN TO HANDLE THE UPCOMING HOLIDAYS

The holiday season happens every year. Miracle-ville.com acted as study participants as we tried on a new plan for the holidays for those on any step of MM. We did not expect weight or inch loss during this time, but we wanted to achieve really enjoyable celebrations. The plan works! Most participants lost a small amount of weight and inches, while others maintained their weight and inches. Great success!

For those who prefer to just stay the course and remain in the MM step they are working in, by all means, carry on. Step One involves tight control and a yes-no attitude that makes it easy to stay the course if you remain focused on your goal. You can bake and freeze Step One cookies just like you would bake regular treats. We have an entire forum dedicated to holiday recipes, most of which match Step One. If you have a slip-up, add three days to the end of your eight weeks and you can stay with Step One right through to New Year's Day!

For those who prefer a little more freedom over the holiday time that precedes New Year's, here is a plan that will work and give you the freedom to participate comfortably in your holidays without significant fallout.

The Plan

November 1 to November 10: Step One

November 11 to day before Thanksgiving: Step Two with no slip-ups

Thanksgiving: Make Thanksgiving dinner your one slip-up for the week! Thoroughly enjoy the holiday but get back on Step Two right afterward for the rest of the day. If you keep nipping on a little stuffing here, a little cranberry sauce there, just one teeny slice of pie, you will spiral backward.

Day after Thanksgiving to December 6: Step One

December 7 to December 23: Step Two with no slip-ups

December 24 to January 1: Step Three for your desired weight

January 2: MM Recommit to Step One for the first eight weeks of the New Year!

8

Rules to Thrive By

As you follow all three steps of the Metabolism Miracle, keep these ten easy Rules to Thrive By in mind. Before you know it, they'll be such a part of your life that you won't even have to think about them.

Rules to Thrive By

1. Drink at least sixty-four ounces of water and other caffeine-free fluids. (Those under five-foot-three need at least forty-eight ounces water or caffeine-free liquids.)
2. Avoid gaps of more than five hours without a meal or snack. Spread your food intake throughout the entire day and even into the night. Within one hour of waking up and one hour before bed, be sure to have a meal or snack.
3. Take the recommended vitamins, minerals, and supplements.
4. Choose nonnutritive sweeteners with care. I recommend the use of Splenda, stevia, or erythritol as sugar substitutes.
5. Judge the carbohydrate content of packaged foods by reading the Nutrition Facts on food labels and using the net carb formula (see page 64).
6. Consider drinking green tea daily.
7. Increase your physical activity to include a minimum of thirty minutes, five times per week, and change it up every eight weeks.
8. Eat neutral foods liberally but not to excess.
9. Practice relaxing. Take a few minutes each day to close your eyes, breathe deeply, shed your stress, and clear your mind.

10. Think positively! First thing in the morning and the last thing at night remind yourself of your good health, weight loss, high energy level, determination, continuing progress, and positive future.

Most of the rules have already been explained in earlier chapters. This chapter will give you more information on why you need to drink at least a half gallon of fluid every day, why you need to spread your food throughout the day, why you should consider drinking green tea, and which supplements you should consider.

Drink Up!

When you're on a fat-burning regimen it is absolutely critical you drink enough decaffeinated fluids. When fat is burned, a buildup of waste products accumulates in the blood and must be cleared from the bloodstream. If you fail to drink adequate fluid, your blood will become overly concentrated with waste products. This waste buildup forces the kidneys to work harder, slows your metabolic rate, and changes the pH of your blood to become more acidic. If you fail to drink enough decaffeinated fluid or water, your body will take fluid from your tissues to help dilute the concentrated blood.

Further, the brain senses the waste buildup in the blood. The brain will intentionally slow fat burning until the blood is properly diluted. As you can see, it's vitally important to drink enough fluids on a fat-burning program or else you will slow your weight loss. I recommend drinking at least sixty-four ounces (a half gallon) of caffeine-free fluids each day. If you are under five-foot-three, you need a minimum of forty-eight ounces fluid intake per day.

Two Quick Ways to Check Your Hydration:
Don't judge your fluid balance by your thirst. After the age of twenty the body's ability to sense dehydration has already begun to diminish. By age seventy there can be little to no warning of your hydration status.

To gauge whether you're drinking enough, use the following two methods.

1. When urine is deep yellow in color, it may be overly concentrated. Check the color of your urine. When you are drinking enough fluids it should be pale yellow in color.
2. Here's an unscientific but trusty indication of your fluid status. Put one hand, palm side down, on a table. Pinch together a little skin from the top of your resting hand and hold the pinch for a count of five. Let the skin go and see how long it takes for the pinched skin to return to normal. A hydrated hand will smooth out quickly; an *under-hydrated* hand will return to normal slowly.

Fluids containing caffeine do not count toward the sixty-four-ounce allotment because caffeine acts as a diuretic, causing you to eliminate more fluid than you have taken in. When you drink twelve ounces of regular coffee, you will urinate more than twelve ounces. This leaves you less hydrated than before you drank the coffee! For this reason do not count any caffeinated beverages toward your daily fluid intake.

Not everyone gets enough mileage out of sixty-four fluid ounces. A large-framed man might need more; a small-framed woman may need less. In any case, drink, drink, and drink some more. It's a great way to care for yourself and one of the easiest things you can do to protect your health and improve your skin, nails, and hair.

If constipation plagues you, take extra precautions to drink enough fluid. The majority of patients who complain of constipation do not drink enough water or decaf fluid throughout the day.

Green Tea

Much of the press about green tea comes from an antioxidant in green tea leaves that is released when the tea steeps. The antioxidant EGCG (epigallocatechin gallate) contained in green tea leaves has been linked to a reduced risk of breast, prostate, colon, and skin cancers; the lowering of LDL cholesterol; and aiding in the breakdown of belly fat. Other studies show green tea might help prevent dental cavities and act as a blood thinner. If you are on blood thinners like Coumadin™ (warfarin), consult your physician before drinking green tea.

I recommend a minimum of two green tea bags per day (many green tea advocates consume at least four green tea bags per day!). Bring water to just before boiling, pour over your teabags, and let it steep for three minutes or more. Consume the tea on the same day it is brewed to ensure its potency. Decaffeinated green tea has less potency than caffeinated green tea; I recommend four decaffeinated green tea bags a day if they are replacing your two green tea bag recommendation.

Some green tea is premade and sold in cans, bottles, or plastic bottles. This tea is not fresh, and although it is green tea, its EGCG is no longer viable. The same principle applies to green tea extracts, concentrates, gum, or pills. Get your EGCG from freshly steeped green tea leaves.

What Beverages Are Allowed?

Pure water should make up the majority of your fluid intake. To keep track, consider drinking your water from bottles or a half-gallon pitcher. When it comes to water, I keep track of the four sixteen-ounce reusable cups I fill per day. When I finish my fourth sixteen-ounce cup, I'm at my goal.

Other good choices include:

- flavored water
- flavored or plain seltzer
- some flavored fitness waters (check label for net carb grams) sweetened with Splenda, stevia, or erythritol
- caffeine-free or herbal tea (hot or iced)
- decaffeinated coffee (hot or iced)
- caffeine-free diet soda (sweetened with Splenda, erythritol, or stevia)
- club soda
- water infused with lemon or lime

Eat Throughout the Day, from Wake-Up Until Bedtime

A popular diet program allots dieters a certain number of points that correspond to the number of calories they may use in the course of the day. According to this plan, as long as the point allotment is used up by the end of the day, the dieter is on track. Another famous diet plan cautions dieters to avoid eating after 6:00 p.m. because evening calories go straight to fat. These popular theories work *against* anyone with Metabolism B. Your weight is not based on the textbook formula that says calories eaten minus calories burned equals body weight.

Those with Metabolism B should spread food throughout the entire day. Eat within one hour of waking up, don't let more than five hours pass without a meal or snack, and end your night with a snack within one hour of bedtime. When you decrease the number of times your liver is called upon to releases glycogen, you have better control of your blood glucose, insulin release, and fat deposits. Those with Met B have to eat to lose weight!

When more than five hours pass without eating your body automatically lowers its metabolic rate. Alternatively, when you spread meals and snacks throughout the day, your body stays in the awake metabolic rate that burns consistently higher. Think of eating from wake-up to bedtime as though you were periodically putting kindling on a fire. If you dump it all on the flames at one time, the fire will burn brightly but burn out quickly. When you instead fuel the fire with the kindling throughout the day and night, the fire will burn steadily. Carbohydrate foods are the kindling for the Metabolism B fire that will burn fat. Eating throughout the day gives the most steady, long-term burn.

Recommended Vitamins, Minerals, and Supplements

I believe that the following supplements help to optimize health throughout life, but they are particularly important during Step One of the Metabolism Miracle, when there is a temporary restriction on dense carbohydrates. They have all been shown to work well with the Metabolism Miracle's goals: long-term fat loss, higher energy, and improved health and well-being. When I work with any of my patients, Met A or Met B, I typically recommend them as insurance that their nutritional needs are being met.

Inform your physician of any supplements you intend to take, and remember to keep a copy of your medications, supplements, and doses in your wallet.

A Daily Multivitamin with Minerals

Dosage: one daily multivitamin with minerals supplement

This supplement provides insurance that you will meet the recommended daily intake of vitamins and minerals. Women of child-bearing age should choose a multivitamin and mineral supplement that contains iron to help replace iron lost during menstruation. Men can choose a formula designed specifically for men. Women in perimenopause or menopause can use multivitamin formulas specifically designed for mature women.

Calcium Supplement

Dosage: 500 to 600 mg taken twice a day

Calcium is best known for helping to strengthen bones and teeth. Calcium is also involved in regulating your heartbeat and hormone secretion. Calcium's functions are such a priority that the body has a built-in mechanism to obtain calcium if you don't have enough in your daily intake. If you fail to ingest adequate calcium through diet or supplements, your body will leech calcium from your bones and teeth, leading to decreased bone density, tooth loss, and even osteopenia or osteoporosis.

Use calcium that is fortified with vitamin D and magnesium for the best absorption. Calcium comes in different forms, including calcium carbonate, which *must* be taken with food, and calcium citrate, which can be taken with or without food.

If you have undergone gastric bypass surgery, confirm that your physician wants you to use calcium citrate, as it does not require stomach acid to metabolize. If you regularly take antacids for gastric reflux or stomach acid reaching the esophagus, choose calcium citrate.

The body can only absorb up to 600 mg of calcium at one time, so it is important to split your daily dose by taking a maximum of 600 mg of calcium at one meal and the other 600 mg of calcium at another.

Check the dosage of your calcium supplements. I have found many calcium supplements that list two pills or capsules as 600 mg. So each supplement has only 300 mg calcium, and you would need four of these to get 1200 mg in a day. Also, don't bother with a calcium supplement that has 1200 mg in each pill or capsule, as you will absorb 600 mg and lose the other 600 mg.

If calcium supplements constipate you, drink more water. You might also start with half the full dosage for the first week and then increase to your full dosage the following week.

If you are using chewable supplements of any kind, be sure to check for net carb grams per supplement. If you don't, you may be consuming 5 grams net carb twice a day when you take your chewable vitamins and supplements. It's better for those with Met B to use a pill or capsule form rather than flavored chews or gummies.

Fish Oil Capsules*
Dosage: 1200 mg per day of DHA and EPA

Fish oil contains eicosapentaenoic acid (EPA) and docosahexaenoic acid (DHA), omega-3 fatty acids that help reduce coronary vascular disease by decreasing triglycerides and blood pressure, decreasing the growth of atherosclerotic plaque, and decreasing the stickiness of blood platelets, thereby helping to thin the blood.

I recommend 1200 mg per day of DHA/EPA for heart-healthy people, and your physician may recommend up to 2400 mg per day for anyone with heart disease.

Unfortunately many fish oil companies are listing the *mg of fish oil* on the label rather than the *mg of EPA/DHA*. A well-known fish oil supplier lists EPA/DHA with ******* where the milligrams should be listed. All they are saying is that the fish oil has some EPA and DHA, but the consumer has no idea how much.

Find a fish oil supplement that clearly displays the milligrams' worth of EPA and DHA. When you know the true EPA/DHA milligrams in each capsule, you know how many capsules you need to take to equal 1200 mg per day.

It is recommended that you eat a portion of fatty fish, such as sardines, albacore tuna, mackerel, or salmon once or twice a week. These fish are high in omega-3 fatty acids.

---

*Consult with your physician before beginning omega 3 supplementation, especially if you have a low platelet level or take a blood thinner such as Warfarin (Coumadin). Excessive intakes may cause bleeding.

WHEN SHOULD YOU TAKE YOUR SUPPLEMENTS?

For optimal effectiveness divide your supplements and take them on a full stomach after two different meals in the day as follows:

With one meal*

- 1 multivitamin with minerals
- 500 to 600 mg of calcium with magnesium and vitamin D_3
- 1000 to 1200 mg of EPA/DHA from fish oil
- 1000 IUs of vitamin D (your physician may recommend more if you are vitamin D deficient)

With another meal

- 500 to 600 mg of calcium with magnesium and vitamin D_3
- 1000 to 1200 mg of EPA/DHA from fish oil
- 1 B-complex vitamin (B-50 or B-100)

---

*People with Met B have a higher incidence of thyroid disease (hypothyroidism). People using thyroid medications like Levoxyl or Synthroid are usually prescribed to take their medication as soon as they awake and then wait thirty to sixty minutes before having breakfast. If you are a thyroid patient, I recommend you take your vitamins and supplements at lunch and at dinner instead of at breakfast and dinner.

B-Complex (B-50)

B vitamins help convert carbohydrates into glucose, which explains why B vitamins are known for providing energy. They also help with metabolizing fat and protein, promote a healthy nervous system, and help beautify skin, hair, and nails. Vitamin B1 helps boost the immune system and strengthen the body under stressful conditions. Vitamin B6 helps produce certain hormones and chemicals in the brain.

Take your B-complex supplement at a meal other than the meal with which you take your multivitamin. B vitamins are water soluble, and if you take both your multivitamin and your B-complex at the same time, you will lose your extra B vitamins to your urine.

B vitamins are effective for approximately twelve hours after ingestion. In order to have adequate B vitamins twenty-four hours a day, I recommend the B-complex as well as the B's in a multivitamin at separate times.

Vitamin D
Dosage: 1000 IUs per day, or as recommended by your physician
Vitamin D, also known as the sunshine vitamin, can be produced in the body with mild sun exposure or consumed in food or supplements. It is estimated that sensible sun exposure on bare skin for fifteen to thirty minutes daily enables the body to produce sufficient vitamin D. Morning sunshine is best. Despite this, recent studies have suggested that up to 50 percent of adults and children worldwide are vitamin D deficient.

Almost everyone with uncontrolled Met B has low vitamin D. Uncontrolled Met B upsets hormonal balance. In spite of the name, vitamin D is not really considered a vitamin but rather a pro-hormone (see Walking on Sunshine, page 107).

Adequate vitamin D intake is important in order to regulate calcium absorption and maintain teeth and bones, and it has been shown to aid in weight loss and decrease the risk of certain cancers, diabetes, and multiple sclerosis.

Planned Slip-Ups:
Intentional Breaks to Help Stay the Course

The Metabolism Miracle is designed to help you reach and maintain permanent weight loss, improved health, and overall well-being. In life there will be special times such as holiday meals, celebrations, vacations, and social gatherings when you make the decision to go off your plan for a meal or a brief time. These little breaks can actually be very helpful for staying the course. I always plan to slip-up at my birthday dinner, my anniversary celebration, certain food-related holidays, and vacation. These are planned slips-ups, and I know exactly how to accommodate them without jeopardizing all the positive things I've accomplished.

On the Metabolism Miracle program planned slip-ups generally fall into two categories.

1. *The party or special occasion "one meal slip-up":* When most traditional dieters plan a celebratory meal, they usually save up calories

during the day and indulge at the party. One popular weight-loss program uses a point system, allotting points to be saved up and placed anywhere in the day. You are now well aware that this system can never work with your body's physiology because your weight is not a function of calories but of the overprocessing of blood glucose into fat cells.

When living the Metabolism Miracle program, if you decide to go off your plan for a celebratory meal, don't change anything during the day to compensate for the "off-meal." Leave your day exactly as it should be up until the party meal, enjoy the party, and then return to your plan that night with the appropriate snack. Metabolism B does not allow you to make up for a slip-up by changing an earlier or later meal to have fewer carbs.

Enjoy your slip-up meal, and then return to your plan. I don't recommend allowing yourself a slip-up more than once a week.

Step One slip-up meal: For every slip-up in a five-hour block on Step One, add three days to the end of your Step One.

Step Two slip-up meal: You are allowed two slip-ups per week on Step Two. I always assume that I have had one slip-up without knowing it during a week on Step Two and allow myself *one planned slip-up per week.* If I have more than two "conscious" slip-ups during a week on Step Two, I do two weeks on Step One to clean the slate so Step Two will continue to allow weight loss and fat burning.

Step Three slip-up meal: It's not often necessary to have a slip-up on Step Three. The maintenance step allows you to shift your carb servings so you can have a greater number of carb servings at one meal as long as your other meals are covered with at least one carb serving. After the holidays or a vacation I often clean up with two weeks of Step One and two weeks of Step Two before returning to Step Three.

A Sample Party Day

7:00 a.m.: Breakfast (with appropriate carb target)

10:30 a.m.: Midmorning snack (with appropriate carb target)

1:00 p.m.: Lunch (with appropriate carb target)

4:00 p.m.: Midafternoon snack (with appropriate carb target)

6:30 p.m.: Party (you're not counting carbs)

11:00 p.m.: Bedtime snack (with appropriate carb target)

2. *The long weekend, holiday, or vacation slip-up:* For a typical dieter it's the excess calories that cause weight gain during a vacation or holiday. For those with Metabolism B weight and fat gain can occur due to excess carb, inadequate carb, improper timing of carb, and/or type of carb. Vacation shakes up your routine, and that means meals may get delayed without Carb Dam snacks, you may sleep in or go to bed late, or you may eat foods whose carbs are higher than you thought.

The best way to handle these extended slip-ups is to reprogram your system once you're home again. As soon as possible upon returning home start a two-week detox on Step One, followed by two weeks of reprogramming with Step Two.

Detox: two weeks of Step One
Reprogram: two weeks of Step Two
Back to Basics: Return to Step Two or Three—whichever step you
    were on prior to your vacation.

I sometimes consider eating out at a restaurant a planned slip-up. This way I can order sensibly from the menu without fretting that the carb probably exceeds my target range. Remember to stay within your carb range right up to and after the out-of-the-ordinary meal. Don't try to make up for excess carbs.

Never fret after a planned slip-up of several days. Remember that *The Metabolism Miracle* is written for you, and you are meant to lead a full and healthful life. You now know how to occasionally accommodate a little food fun without negative repercussions. The trick is to plan for the slip-up and also plan for the cleanup afterward. Move forward in a positive direction, don't wallow in guilt, and get back on track so you can continue to reap all the benefits of your new and improved life.

You'll soon follow the Rules to Thrive By so well that they'll become a part of your life, just as a child learns to ride a bike and never forgets.

9

Exercise Is Half of the Metabolism Miracle Program

You don't need a gym membership, expensive equipment, or a personal trainer for the exercise portion of the Metabolism Miracle. All you need is a minimum of thirty minutes a day over and above your usual activity. These thirty minutes needn't be carved out of your day in one block; you can do the thirty minutes in mini-blocks throughout the day.

I have found that people are willing to "do the diet" but are not so willing to "do the exercise." On the Metabolism Miracle, exercise is half the program. If you follow your diet guidelines to the letter but don't get physically active, you will not reap the benefits of this amazing program. I tell my patients, "If you follow the diet but don't exercise, you will only get half the results—because you skipped half the MM program when you didn't exercise."

Keep in mind that in the case of Metabolism B, your weight is *not* entirely the result of eating more calories than you burn. Your weight is mainly a function of progressive insulin imbalance and insulin resistance that led to fat cell overgrowth.

Exercise works to stimulate muscle cells to burn more blood glucose. Less insulin is needed for lower blood glucose. Exercise is a "nonmedicine" medicine for fat burning and muscle retention. In addition, physical activity tones your muscles and helps direct your body to focus on burning fat.

When you exercise as prescribed, you will retain a great shape as you burn the fat that has covered your muscles, stoke your metabolic rate, improve your mood, increase your energy, and relieve stress. If a pill could do all of this, you'd pay a fortune for it. Exercise is half the Metabolism Miracle—for good reason!

Make It Burn

Your goal is to burn fat and retain muscle. If you've been sitting around for the past months or years doing little more than walking from the house to the car and from the parking lot to your office, your muscle has been relatively inactive. Your metabolism is switched on low. You feel lethargic, unmotivated, melancholy, and weak.

Imagine that your fat tissue *and inactive* muscle tissue appeared dark blue in color. The brain would not be able to distinguish between the two types of tissue and could choose to burn either fat or muscle when seeking energy while carb intake is low.

When you get off the couch for a regular evening walk, exercise activates the muscle tissue. Think of activated muscle tissue changing from dark blue to bright red. The brain can easily distinguish between the two and will choose to burn the fat tissue, leaving the beneficial muscle intact.

Muscle is metabolically active tissue. Once stimulated, it burns calories for hours after the workout. The more muscle tissue, the more "furnaces," and the more efficiently your body handles blood glucose. Fat's main functions, however, are to insulate the body and to provide a stockpile of calories for times of famine. Fat is not metabolically active and does not burn calories at rest.

As long as you have exercised in tandem with the Metabolism Miracle diet, your brain can clearly differentiate between muscle and fat tissue—and will choose to burn the fat and retain the muscle. If, however, you decide to remain sedentary, the brain will burn both fat and muscle tissue. You will lose weight, but along with the fat you hoped to lose, you will also lose valuable muscle.

There's No Getting Away from It—You MUST Exercise on MM!

I once had a patient with Metabolism B who followed the Miracle program with his wife. He exercised faithfully for thirty minutes, five times a week, but she opted not to exercise. When they returned in eight weeks for a follow-up, the wife had lost more weight on the scale than her husband. Unfortunately the wife reported feeling a little weak, fatigued, and complained of vague aches and pains.

Her exercising husband looked as if he had lost far more weight than his spouse had. He had trimmed five inches off his waist, looked slimmer, and felt more energized. In addition, his lab work showed impressive decreases in cholesterol, triglycerides, glucose, and blood pressure.

As she gloated about her greater weight loss, I had to explain that without exercising, her brain had been directing her body to burn both muscle and fat tissue.

Muscle, the heavier tissue, showed up as more weight loss. As she lost muscle tissue, the woman also lost valuable furnaces for burning fat. Her husband, who burned all fat tissue as he retained muscle, looked like a much thinner and younger man.

Remember, when you finish losing your excess fat and have found your desired weight and size, you will appear ten to fifteen pounds thinner than your scale weight because you burned the fat and retained the muscle. Go you!

How Much and What Kind of Exercise Do I Need?

To retain muscle tissue and burn fat tissue, you need to increase your physical activity over and above your own personal norm. You will need a minimum of thirty minutes of increased activity for a minimum of five days per week. You need to change up your activity by increasing

RAYMOND, THE FRUSTRATED EXERCISER

Raymond, an automotive mechanic and overall nice guy, had a stubborn roll of fat around his belly and felt out of shape, fatigued, and older than his fifty-nine years. He was five-foot-ten and now weighed 202 pounds. Because his job as a mechanic was physical, he never thought he needed to exercise. But as the years progressed, so too did his belly's size.

To "whoop him into shape," Ray got in touch with his longtime friend, the high school football coach, Elio G. This guy was "old school." He soon had Raymond on an exercise program including weight lifting, running, the "medicine ball," and speed drills.

Basically Ray was now in boot camp, attempting to do the same program the teen athletes did to get in shape before football season.

Ray took the regimen seriously. He did all the exercises—one hour a day, five days a week—at his own pace. But he was putting in five grueling hours a week.

Several weeks passed, and Ray's side profile as well as the weight on the scale did not budge. Elio explained that muscle weighs more than fat and that Ray might not immediately see weight loss as he was rebuilding muscle. Ray wondered, Where the heck is this muscle? It appeared as if a coating of fat covered up all his hard work. There was no sign of muscle and no loss of his belly despite Elio's crazy, old-school, intense workout.

Eventually Coach Elio, who came to realize that Ray had not made any healthy changes with his diet, referred his friend to my office for evaluation, saying, "It is impossible for Ray to eat the amount of food that he reports, to work out to the degree he has been, and still have no significant results."

the duration, speed, weights, or types of activity to keep the muscles motivated.

If your daily job or lifestyle contains built-in activity, like that of a waiter, construction worker, nurse, or mother of twin toddlers, your body has come to expect this level of daily activity. This is your norm. You'll need to add thirty minutes of activity to your day for the muscle activation that MM requires.

Some Metabolism B dieters wonder whether instead of five days for thirty minutes, they can do two and a half hours of exercise all in one

It turns out that Ray's latest fasting blood glucose was 102 mg/dL, indicative of prediabetes. His doctor had already circled his LDL cholesterol, triglycerides, and blood pressure as high. He also had low vitamin D and low HDL (good) cholesterol. The fasting lab work confirmed that Ray had uncontrolled Metabolism B.

Ray walked into my office without making eye contact and said, "You are my last hope. I am watching everything I eat, exercising my backside off, and I can't lose inches or pounds. My labs and blood pressure are off, and I feel wiped out, depressed, and irritable with my grandkids."

Sure enough, his food log proved that Ray was eating the calories of a man of his age and height weighing 172 pounds.

I taught Ray all about Met B and the Metabolism Miracle program. We did discuss Fueling Forward for Ray's one hour of exercise on Step One. He would take 11- to 20-gram quick carbs at the start of exercise and at the thirty-minute mark and end with a protein source.

Within a few weeks of starting the Metabolism Miracle program, with Coach Elio's old-school workout plan, Ray began to see the difference in his body. He kept up with his exercise program, but this time, as he burned fat, his muscles showed tone and form. He also lost weight for the first time in months. Even better, he regained his energy and felt brighter and calmer.

By his next physical exam Ray's lab work had returned to normal. He's been on the maintenance phase of the Metabolism Miracle since he reached his desired weight and size, and he says, "MM is not a diet. MM plus Coach Elio are my new way of life."

day. It's a nice concept, but your muscle tissue needs regular stimulation so your brain will target fat cells on a daily basis. One day of activity will burn fat for that day but will not direct the brain for the next day. If you move your muscles throughout the course of the week, your brain will consistently choose to burn fat tissue. Exercising activates living muscle and increases your metabolism. A sedentary life does not preserve muscle and allows it to be burned along with fat.

The type of physical activity you choose is up to you. Mix it up to stimulate different muscle groups and to keep your interest. Walking, swimming, gardening, biking, yoga, light weight lifting, weight train-ing, skiing, snow shoveling, tennis, using gym machines such as a treadmill or elliptical, aerobic exercise, spinning, and Zumba all stim-ulate muscle tissue (see Twenty-One Easy Ways to Start Moving, on the opposite page).

If your mobility is restricted, ask your physician about armchair ex-ercises; exercising while in a chair might work for you. Many patients lift light weights or do leg lifts while watching television. If you pick up a two-pound weight and lift it during commercials, putting it down when the program returns and then shifting arms for the next batch of commercials, you can easily activate muscle tissue for thirty minutes without leaving your chair during the course of a two-hour television movie.

If you are recovering from an injury or accident, your physical ther-apy counts as your exercise time. You needn't gasp for air or sweat like there's no tomorrow to have a workout; you simply need a min-imum of thirty minutes over and above your typical activity for five days/week. This thirty minutes may be broken into three ten-minute intervals.

Every eight weeks change up your exercise—its speed, duration, or type of activity—to keep muscle tissue "interested" and not complacent with the same old, same old. You raised the exercise bar eight weeks pre-vious, but that exercise has now become your new norm.

To change up your exercise routine:

- Add another few minutes to your routine.
- Elevate the treadmill to the next height.
- Add more tension to your elliptical.
- Increase the speed of your workout.
- Add a little more weight to your light weights.
- Mix up your exercise choices, like in circuit training.

Some people leave the thirty minutes intact but increase the pace. Each subtle change reinvigorates the body and keeps your exercise out of the norm for your body. Dance like no one's watching or walk an extra block. Never stagnate; always move forward.

TWENTY-ONE EASY WAYS TO START MOVING

1. Take a brisk ten-minute walk before work, a fifteen-minute walk at lunch, and a ten-minute walk before you go home. When you go home at the end of the day you are done!
2. During two hours of television programming, instead of fast forwarding or munching through the thirty minutes of commercials, lift hand weights, do calisthenics, march in place, or climb the stairs several times.
3. Work in your garden.
4. Mow your lawn with a walking mower.
5. Take a yoga or tai chi class.
6. Clean out the garage.
7. Wash the floors—the old-fashioned way.
8. Wash your car by hand.
9. Ride your bike or walk to get the morning paper or go to the post office.
10. Work out to a thirty-minute exercise video.
11. Take an after-dinner walk with your family or brisk walk at the mall with a friend.
12. Pace the sidelines during your child's athletic games or walk the track before the game begins.
13. Bike to the park and back.
14. Swim, play tennis, or play golf (without the golf cart).
15. Take a hike (I say this with love).
16. Walk your dog.
17. Take the stairs instead of the elevator.
18. Play tag, jump rope, play basketball, or try the hula hoop or scooter with your children for at least thirty minutes a day.
19. While on a conference call walk during the conversation or lift light weights at your desk.
20. Turn on your favorite music and dance.
21. Wear a pedometer and compete with a friend to see who walks the most steps per day over a month's time.

The timing of exercise makes a difference for people with Metabolism B. You will benefit the most if you schedule exercise in relation to your meals and snacks. These simple guidelines will maximize your fat burning by complementing your metabolic system. If the same amount and type of activity is placed at the right time, you can increase its benefit.

If you work out first thing in the morning, start with a pre-exercise snack.
As you already know, when you first awaken your body is still functioning with the help of glycogen released every five hours by the liver. If you wake up and exercise without shutting the liver's self-feeding mechanism off, your liver will continue to release sugar throughout your exercise routine and afterward. That will stimulate your pancreas to over-release insulin, open more fat cells, and cause fat gain. You could be exercising in the morning and promoting weight gain!

For the most efficient workout, exercise between one and two hours after the start of a meal.
Your blood glucose peaks about two hours after you begin to eat. If you time your activity for this peak period, the muscles activated during your exercise session will burn blood glucose from the food and suppress excess insulin release and fat storage.

Take a snack before exercise if it's been four or more hours since you've last eaten. On Step One exercise lasting forty minutes or more allows you to Fuel Forward.
During Steps Two and Three, if four or more hours have passed since you last ate, it is best to take a pre-exercise snack, as you have exceeded five hours without an 11- to 20-gram Carb Dam or carb serving.

Fueling Forward

When exercising for long periods of time you should Fuel Forward (FF) to feed your muscles the energy they need. With Fueling Forward, you should notice lots of energy during your workout and no fatigue, aches, or ravenous appetite when you finish exercise. Each FF quick-carb selection fuels the upcoming thirty minutes of exercise, and protein after the workout helps to rebuild and retain muscle tissue.

Fuel Forward carb choices include:

- 3 to 4 glucose tablets (found over the counter at your pharmacy or supermarket pharmacy section)
- Carb gel in a portion that contains 11 to 20 grams net carb
- 3 Gatorade Chews™
- 1 serving of Step Two fruit
- 1 tablespoon of honey
- ½ cup of juice (you may dilute with water)
- ½ cup of regular Jell-O™

Fueling Forward on Step One

After the fifth day of Step One your liver and muscles have been purposely depleted of glycogen stores. On Step One, within ten minutes before exercise that will last forty or more minutes, you should take a fast-acting carb choice. (This is not a 5-gram Counter Carb; it is 11 to 20 grams of quick carbohydrate that will fuel your thirty minutes of exercise and burn off by the end of thirty minutes.)

After taking your Fueling Forward source, exercise for forty minutes. If you intend to exercise for one hour, take your first quick-carb choice within ten minutes of starting to exercise and take another quick-carb selection to fuel the upcoming thirty minutes.

If your exercise will continue past the one-hour mark, take another quick-carb selection at the one-hour mark to fuel the upcoming thirty minutes. Total exercise would now equal ninety minutes, and you would have consumed three Fueling Forward quick carbs: before exercise, at the thirty-minute mark, and at the sixty-minute mark. You fueled the entire ninety-minute workout!

Within thirty minutes after finishing exercise have a protein source. This protein may be a string cheese, a spoon of natural peanut butter, or a low-carb protein shake.

Example of Fueling Forward for Step One

6:00 a.m.: Wake up

6:15 a.m.: Breakfast with 5-gram Counter Carb

7:30 a.m. to 9:30 a.m.: Bike race: because the race will last two hours, there will be Fueling Forward for every upcoming thirty-minute period:

7:30 a.m.: Take your initial 11- to 20-gram quick carb.

8:00 a.m.: Take another 11- to 20-gram quick carb.

8:30 a.m.: Take another 11- to 20-gram quick carb.

9:00 a.m.: Take another 11- to 20-gram quick carb.

9:30 a.m.: Within thirty minutes of completing the race have some protein such as a cheese stick, a spoonful of natural peanut butter, or a low-carb protein shake.

On Steps Two or Three

When on Steps Two or Three you only need to Fuel Forward *after* the first hour of long-duration exercise is complete. Take your 11- to 20-gram quick-acting carb at the end of hour one and every half-hour thereafter.

Many people do not Fuel Forward on Steps Two and Three, but long workouts (over one hour in duration) can benefit from Fueling Forward after the one-hour mark by keeping the metabolic rate high and fueling duration exercise and are totally burned off over the next thirty minutes of muscle stimulation.

Example of Fueling Forward for Steps Two and Three

6:00 a.m.: Wake up

6:45 a.m.: Breakfast with 11 to 20 grams net carb

7:30 a.m. until 9:30 a.m.: Bike ride that will last two hours. For the first hour of the race no Fueling Forward is necessary.

8:30 a.m.: Take an 11- to 20-gram quick carb, such as 3 Gatorade Chews or glucose tablets.

9:00 a.m.: Take another 11- to 20-gram quick carb, such as 3 Gatorade Chews or glucose tablets. These will cover your activity through the end of the race.

9:30 a.m.: Within thirty minutes of completing the race have some protein such as a cheese stick, a spoonful of natural peanut butter, or a low-carb protein shake.

Keep a log of your exercise in a prominent place, such as on the refrigerator. It will help you see your progress and remind you when you need to set aside thirty minutes for more activity.

Use the chart on page 194 to start your record. When you complete thirty minutes put a check in the box. If you add extra minutes, jot them next to the thirty-minute checkmark. Five checkmarks are needed per week.

Treat the squares on this chart like the sections of a pillbox. You wouldn't skip taking your blood pressure medication, so don't skip taking your exercise. It's the critical link for anyone on the Metabolism Miracle program.

Frequently Asked Questions About Exercise

I don't have a thirty-minute block of time in which to exercise. Is it ok to do less?

You don't have to exercise for thirty minutes in succession. The idea is to energize your muscles for at least thirty minutes above and beyond your normal level of activity, five days per week. It's fine to get your exercise in intervals: fifteen minutes or more in the morning, fifteen minutes or more in the evening. You can even consider ten-minute intervals three times a day.

I want to lose as much weight as possible. By skipping the exercise, I enable my body to burn both muscle and fat and lose more pounds on the scale. I'm going to skip the exercise.

Stop! It's true that if you were to follow the diet part of MM without exercising, you might lose more weight on the scale. But you will lose valuable muscle along with your fat, lower your metabolic rate, and lose many muscle furnaces as muscles are burned for energy. You might lose more weight (muscle weight), but you will not look much smaller.

After day five of Step One your brain will choose to burn either fat or muscle tissue. Daily exercise steers your brain to burn fat, which is big

Month _____

Monthly Exercise Log

	Monday	Tuesday	Wednesday	Thursday	Friday	Saturday	Sunday	days/week
WEEK ONE								
WEEK TWO								
WEEK THREE								
WEEK FOUR								

Put a check in the box if you've exercised more than thirty minutes that day.

and fluffy tissue that makes you look puffy, bloated, jiggly, and emphasizes rolls and bulges. When you don't exercise, your body will *also* burn muscle, the heavy dense tissue that gives you firmness, shape, and tone. Muscle also helps burn blood glucose and decreases insulin production.

I've heard that to get any health benefit from exercise, there must be a warm-up, at least thirty minutes of cardio, and then a cool-down. Your program seems much easier. Will I really get a workout and lose weight with this program?

The answer depends on what you want to achieve. It takes at least thirty minutes of aerobic activity at your target heart rate to get cardio benefits. Weight lifting helps tone muscles and maintain bone mass and fits the Metabolism Miracle requirement of thirty minutes a day, five times a week. But weight lifting doesn't get your heart rate into the cardio zone. Gardening requires muscle stimulation and also fits the Miracle requirement but probably won't get you to the cardio level. Running for thirty minutes achieves better cardio health and a trimmer, toned physique.

I cannot imagine eating a snack before I exercise in the morning. I want to burn my excess fat and don't want a Fueling Forward snack to slow down my weight-loss progress.

If you exercise while on Step One for more than forty minutes continuously, you should consider Fueling Forward as a way to give you energy for a great workout and help eliminate aches, pains, and muscle burn as well as prevent fatigue later in the day. On Steps Two or Three you need to Fuel Forward after the first hour of exercise. The 11- to 20-gram quick-carb choice fuels the energy needed for thirty minutes and is burned away. There is no residual left in the bloodstream after the workout. The snack goes in, fuels the activity, and is gone.

In the not-too-distant past, duration exercisers like tri-athletes, marathoners, distance swimmers, and bicyclers would go very low carb before a race or long training and then "carb load" during the meal before the exercise. The problem with this technique is that this high intake of carb grams causes a rapid rise in blood sugar and insulin gush from the pancreas, so those with Met B won't improve their stamina this way. Met B duration exercisers will run out of energy and feel wiped out faster than if they Fueled Forward for each upcoming thirty-minute interval. So on Step Two or Three, after one hour of activity, take an 11- to 20-gram quick carb and repeat at the end of the half-hour to fuel the upcoming thirty minutes. After the exercise have some protein (e.g., a meal with lots of protein, a low-carb protein shake, some cheese, a spoonful of natural peanut butter, eggs, etc.).

Can I use 11 to 20 grams of net carb from chocolate, pudding, or ice cream to Fuel Forward?

The carbohydrate you use to Fuel Forward (FF) must consist of quick carbohydrate only. The fat and protein in other foods will prevent the carb grams from entering your blood and cause a blood sugar rise *after* exercise is done.

You'll notice that FF choices are composed of sugar: honey, carb gel, juice, fruit from Step Two, and glucose tabs, among others. When you consume these, they cause a rise in blood glucose that your muscles will burn for fuel and are quickly out of your bloodstream. You will have no weight gain, but you will have a *great* workout, stronger muscles, and a toned body—all great reasons to Fuel Forward for exercise that lasts forty minutes or more.

I understand the need to block the liver while I'm exercising. What if I exercise two or three hours after a meal—do I still need that pre-exercise snack?

Examples:

6:00 p.m.: Dinner
8:00 p.m.: Exercise requires *no snack*

BUT

1:00 p.m.: Lunch
5:00 p.m.: Exercise *requires* an 11- to 20-gram net carb snack, as you
    will finish exercise four hours or more since you last ate.

Two hours after breakfast I like to bike. If the ride lasts two hours, should I snack afterward so as not to go too long between meals?

Absolutely. Don't go more than five hours between meals, regardless of whether you are active during that time. Because it is two hours of exercise, you would Fuel Forward from the start for every half-hour if on Step One or wait until the first hour of exercise is done before Fueling Forward for the upcoming thirty-minute blocks of exercise.

10

Measuring Up

How to Monitor Your Progress
Without Daily or Weekly Weigh-Ins

Weigh yourself in the morning on the day you begin the program. Accurately obtain body measurements on this day too. Take all the body measurements indicated on page 202. Then save your data, hide the measuring tape and scale, and begin following MM like it's your job.

During those first eight weeks your body will adjust to an entirely new way of burning fat that involves the normalization of your blood glucose and insulin release. You will see your progress in your lab work, weight, and inches *after* you finish any eight-week block, with days added for slip-ups, of Steps One and Two of the MM program.

Those living the MM lifestyle lose weight when their insulin is balanced and normalized. On MM you focus on carb control: keeping track of the amount, type, and timing of carbs *and* purposeful exercise over and above your normal physical activity.

The Metabolism Miracle Is Not a Calorie-Counting Program—
MM Is a Carb-Centric, Insulin-Normalizing Program

Low-calorie programs promise one to two pounds' loss per week. A pictorial of weight loss for Met A's following a traditional low-calorie diet would resemble a flight of stairs: lose one to two pounds, hang out there for a bit, lose another one to two pounds, and hang out there a bit.

Those with Met B have a whole different story. At some point in the progression of Met B, calorie-based diets cease to work and can actually cause weight gain. Over their lifetime Met B's lose and regain hundreds of pounds as they try to follow diets written for people with Metabolism A.

The scale is the traditional gadget to track progress on a typical weight-loss diet that emphasizes limiting and burning calories. So dieters dutifully weigh themselves every day, coming away with a number that can lift them high or plunge them into despair.

I sometimes think of the bathroom scale as an instrument of torture. Some of my patients admit to weighing themselves as often as three times a day. They remove earrings, watches, wallets, keys, and shoes before stepping on the scale. About one-third of my patients close their eyes during their weigh-in, and some face backward to avoid seeing the number on the scale. Whether they compulsively weigh-in or despise seeing their weight, the number on the scale is a source of great anxiety.

For those with Metabolism B, stepping on a scale on a regular basis (daily/weekly) is *not* recommended as an accurate measure of progress. Most of a Met B's excess weight comes in the form of belly fat and is the result of the body overprocessing carbohydrate into fat as a result of a hormonal imbalance of insulin. Met B weight loss will have dips and pauses that can frustrate you. If you insist on a day-to-day weigh-in to measure your progress, please remember the scale is not your friend.

People assume that when they are "on a diet" their weight will gradually decrease. In reality, if you weigh daily, one of three weight-loss patterns will emerge. Each pattern, shown below, shows a very different outcome and can tell you a lot about your metabolism and health.

The Staircase (Metabolism A)

This type of *plateau weight loss* is the norm and typifies weight loss for people with Metabolism A who follow traditional low-calorie diets. The graph resembles a set of stairs with a few days of weight loss followed by a few days without loss. While you are on the plateau, weight loss temporarily slows or stops for days or even a week. Plateaus often cause dieters to abandon their program.

In actuality the staircase with plateaus is a healthy weight-loss pattern. It occurs when the brain, working like a sensor, detects weight loss and slows the loss until it can assess all of your bodily functions. Once it ascertains that you are healthy, it will allow further weight loss until the next check. In this way the brain can slow starvation or allow healthy weight loss.

The Ski Slope

This pattern represents *uncontrolled weight loss*. Starting weight is the top of the slope, and it continues to decline, uninterrupted. Although this is the type of weight loss most people seek, they don't realize that unchecked weight loss is *not* normal. It often indicates a medical concern such as hyperthyroidism, uncontrolled diabetes, cancer, or gastrointestinal conditions, and it should be a big red flag for healthcare providers.

The Descending Curlicue (Metabolism B)

The weight loss of people with Metabolism B is *hormone mediated*. You will not experience weight loss in nice, neat, predictable steps but rather in a very erratic pattern that occasionally shows you gaining weight! Because of this erratic pattern I recommend weighing and measuring yourself only after your eight weeks on Step One and at the start and finish of eight-week periods thereafter. Note your starting weight and get good body measurements, record and put them in a safe place, go to your book and find your expected fat/inch loss for this eight-week period, and jot it down with the measurement. At the end of eight weeks, with time added for slip-ups, it's time to weigh and remeasure. You should be thrilled with your progress and land within your expected weight and inch loss, with pounds and total inches lost within two or so points of each other. The curlicue weight loss during the eight weeks doesn't matter as long as you end the eight-week block within your expected range.

Trust Your Measuring Tape

In lieu of frequent scale weighing, we will rely on several objective markers to evaluate our progress. These markers should be checked at the start of every eight-week period and at its end. Compare your beginning and ending weight and your beginning and ending measurements, and note if your inches lost and pounds lost are close to a match. You can also check your lab work periodically, note medication changes (lessening or eliminating), and note if your beginning Met B symptoms have disappeared.

Most people are measured by a spouse, partner, friend, older child, or gym assistant. The person who initially measures should be the same person who repeats the same measurements each time, as everyone has his or her own touch with a measuring tape.

Keep a log with eight-week measurements to see your progress, comparing the start of every eight weeks to the end of eight weeks from start to finish.

What's Wrong with Ideal Body Weight Charts and BMI?

The "ideal body weight" charts, once published by life insurance companies, make no distinction between the weight of fat tissue and the weight of muscle tissue. Scale weight is the sum total of all the components of the body, including fat, muscle, bones, fluids, organs, skin, implants, and so forth. Some people who are heavier on the scale or weight chart have less fat and are in much better shape and health than those who don't exercise, have less muscle, more fat, and less body fluid.

	Start of first 8 weeks	End of 8 weeks	End of 8 weeks	End of 8 weeks
Areas to Measure	Step _____ begins Date: _____	Step _____ Date: _____	Step _____ Date: _____	Step _____ Date: _____
Neck				
Chest (fullest area)				
Women (bra line)				
Waistline Belly (largest area)				
Hips (fullest area)				
Right thigh				
Left thigh				
Right calf (midway between knee and ankle)				
Left calf				
Right ankle				
Left ankle				
Right upper arm (midway between elbow and shoulder)				
Left upper arm				
Right wrist				
Left wrist				
INCHES	Total inches:	Total inches: Total inches lost over 8 weeks:	Total inches: Total inches lost over 8 weeks:	Total inches: Total inches lost over 8 weeks:
WEIGHT	Weight:	Weight: Weight lost over 8 weeks:	Weight: Weight lost over 8 weeks:	Weight: Weight lost over 8 weeks:

	Mike	Steven
Age	52	52
Height	6'0"	6'0"
Frame	medium	medium
Weight	180 lbs	160 lbs
Waist	34	37
LDL cholesterol	97	128
Blood pressure	120/72	142/92
Exercise	more than 30 minutes per day, 5 times a week	none

Take a minute to compare the statistics of two men. Ideal body weight charts take into account a person's age, height, weight, *and* frame. By the numbers alone, you would conclude that Steven is in better shape than Mike.

Look a little deeper at their respective waist measurement, cholesterol, LDL cholesterol, blood pressure, and activity level, and you will come to a very different conclusion.

The ideal body weight for a fifty-two-year-old male who is six feet tall and of medium frame is 157 to 170 pounds. Mike is much healthier and leaner than Steve, but he weighs 10 pounds over his ideal body weight. Steve weighs 20 pounds less than Mike and is in his ideal weight range but has a much higher percentage of body fat, less heavy muscle, and unhealthy weight-related lab work and blood pressure.

Another chart system, the BMI (body mass index), has been touted as a more accurate assessment of weight than ideal body weight charts. BMI is a person's weight in kilograms divided by the square of height in meters.

BMI	Weight Status
Below 18.5	Underweight
18.5 to 24.9	Normal or healthy weight
25.0 to 29.9	Overweight
30.0 and above	Obese

Note: BMI chart from CDC (Centers for Disease Control), "Body Mass Index (BMI)," www.cdc.gov/healthyweight/assessing/bmi.

Like the ideal body weight chart, the BMI concept has major flaws. BMI does not distinguish between gender, age, or physical activity level. Instead, it tosses everyone into the same pot, comparing men and women, young and old, active and inactive.

Using the BMI's simple comparison of weight to height, you would use the same chart to find the BMI of a young male athlete and an elderly woman!

Lucky Seven

These seven measures, looked at collectively, are an excellent way to measure MM progress. Check these results every eight weeks of Step One and Two.

1. Total inches lost: Check difference between total inches at the start and total inches eight weeks afterward (plus time added for slip-ups).
2. Loss of pounds: Check difference between total pounds lost by comparing starting weight and eight weeks into the program. (Comparison of inches lost to pounds lost should be within two to three points of each other.)
3. Improvement in your previously uncontrolled Met B symptoms (see page 32–33).
4. Decrease in blood glucose (if previously elevated).
5. Decrease in blood lipids (if previously elevated).
6. Decrease in blood pressure (if previously elevated).
7. Increase in vitamin D level (if previously low).

Starting Too High

Many people begin MM with high levels of glucose and/or lipids (fats) in their blood. Very high glucose and lipid levels will initially alter the speed of the weight loss and fat burning. If you are beginning the Metabolism Miracle with any of the following conditions, please read on.

Uncontrolled type 2 diabetes with very elevated blood glucose. People with diabetes or prediabetes are usually familiar with the lab tests fasting blood glucose and hemoglobin A1C (also known as HbA1C or A1C). Fasting blood glucose gives a reading for that one moment in time, whereas hemoglobin A1C is indicative of your average blood sugar 24/7 for about three months before the test. Hemoglobin A1C is usually drawn quarterly if you have uncontrolled diabetes.

If you begin the Metabolism Miracle with HbA1C between 6.0 and 7.0, your body will spend the first few weeks of MM burning off the excess

WHAT IS YOUR DESIRABLE HEALTHY WEIGHT?

Not a day passes in my weight-loss practice without someone asking, "What is my ideal weight?" I define desired weight as your scale weight when the following happen:

1. Your Met B lab work and blood pressure is in the normal range, with as little medication as possible.
2. You like the way you look and feel. You like how you look in this size of clothing. You are comfortable with your body.
3. You have lots of energy, focus, ability to concentrate, and look and feel younger than you did before the program.

I never use the term "ideal body weight"; I prefer the term "desirable healthy body weight." You won't find it on a chart or in a table, but you will find it in your improved lab work, scale weight, on the measuring tape, and in the way you look and feel. When it's all in order look at the scale. This is your desirable healthy body weight!

When you reach your desirable healthy body weight, you are ready to move to Step Three, the maintenance step of the Metabolism Miracle.

sugar in your bloodstream. If your starting HbA1C is 7.0 or over, it will take even longer before your body begins to burn fat stores. Look at your HbA1C at the start of the program. At your next A1C test you will see a marked drop in A1C, and as your blood sugar normalizes, your A1C will also decrease.

For every point your A1C decreases during Step One or Step Two, you gain and then burn five pounds. This is not crazy math; it is the reality of normalizing A1C without medications!

Someone *without* diabetes or elevated A1C does not gain fat from excess glucose being forced into fat cells. For a nondiabetic, MM simply enables them to burn fat. So they end their eight weeks with their lost weight, inches on target, and in their expected fat- and inch-loss zone.

If you do not have diabetes or you have excellent control of your diabetes (HbA1C less than 6.0), there will be no excess sugar to consume and body fat burning will begin immediately after day five of Step One.

JEAN-ANNE'S "INVISIBLE" WEIGHT LOSS

Jean-Anne has type 2 diabetes and had an A1C of 10.0 when she began the Metabolism Miracle program. When her HbA1C was next checked, she was thrilled to see her A1C had dropped 4 points using the program, coming down to an all-time low of 6.0.

Jean-Anne was thrilled with her new A1C and realized she had made that terrific improvement in blood glucose with the MM program, as her medication actually decreased. When she got on the scale at the end of eight weeks, however, she found that she didn't lose within her target range—she had only lost one pound! Understandably, Jean-Anne was very disappointed in her lower-than-target weight loss. "I was supposed to lose fourteen to twenty-one pounds, and I only lost one pound," she said.

I had to remind her that she began MM with high blood glucose and that this elevated sugar doesn't simply disappear; it is ushered into fat cells, so fat was gained and simultaneously burned with the MM program.

Each point of A1C decrease is actually five pounds of weight being gained and lost. So Jean-Anne's four-point decrease in A1C (4 points x 5 pounds) means she actually lost the twenty pounds she simultaneously gained as her blood glucose normalized.

If Jean Anne simply took medication to lower blood glucose and did not follow MM, she could attain normal blood sugar through the action of the medication, but she would have gained twenty pounds in the process.

So I explained to her that when her A1C dropped four points, she had gained and lost twenty pounds. Instead of her disappointment in losing only one pound, she should see that she had actually lost twenty-one pounds: one pound on the scale plus twenty pounds of fat that was assimilated and then burned when she normalized her A1C by four points.

I also told her that now that she had a fantastic A1C, her next eight weeks would show all the fat burning on the scale. Sure enough, after eight more weeks of Step One she lost twenty-one pounds and twenty-one inches!

High Cholesterol or High Triglycerides

If you start the Metabolism Miracle with elevated LDL cholesterol or triglycerides, your body will consume this excess fat in the beginning of Step One. Once your body has finished burning those blood lipids, it will focus on burning fat cells as you lose inches around your midline and other parts of your body.

If your lipids are in the normal range when you begin the program, fat burning will begin immediately after day five of Step One.

11

Vegetarianism, Gluten Intolerance, Dining Out, and Healthy Shopping

Everyone has personal preferences concerning food. I've worked with many "meat and potato" folks in my practice, but I've also seen a good number of vegetarians as well as those who eat out more often than not. These folks usually express concerns that they won't be able to live the Metabolism Miracle. Nothing could be further from the truth.

Vegetarian Fare

There are different levels of vegetarianism.

An *ovo-lacto vegetarian* (or *lacto-ovo vegetarian*) does not eat any meat, fish, or poultry. But most ovo-lacto vegetarian diets include fruit, vegetables, grains, legumes, nuts, seeds, eggs and egg products, and milk and dairy foods.

On the other end of the spectrum is the strictest vegetarian, the vegan. Vegans exclude all animal products, including dairy and honey. Vegans promote nonanimal alternatives to the consumption or use of animals.

Most vegetarian diets tend to be high in carbohydrate foods, as the base of a vegetarian diet is often composed of carbs such as fruit; grains including bread, bread products, whole-grain pasta, brown rice, and crackers; legumes like chickpeas, hummus, lentils; and starchy vegetables like sweet potatoes, potatoes, and corn.

JOSEPH: NEW TO VEGETARIANISM . . .
AND GAINING WEIGHT?

Joseph, a twenty-six-year-old supermarket manager, recently decided to become a vegetarian because he thought by eliminating meats and meat-based fats he would decrease his calories and lose some weight. Right after college graduation his stress level quadrupled with the responsibilities of paying off college debt and managing a high-volume store. Joseph eliminated meat, fish, and poultry but still consumed egg whites and low-fat dairy. "How many eggs and pieces of cheese can you eat before going crazy?" he asked. To add insult to injury, he actually began to gain weight on his vegetarian program.

I was happy Joe brought a detailed one-week food log to our initial session. Each day contained meals and snacks of whole-grain bread, multi-grain pasta, brown rice, legumes, fruit, fresh-squeezed juice, egg whites, and low-fat cheese, milk, and other dairy products.

I had also seen his latest fasting lab work. His blood pressure was "borderline high," and he was surprised to see that his cholesterol had actually risen on his low-fat, vegetarian program. Joseph had Metabolism B.

He asked me to configure his caloric intake, as he felt that what he was eating did not add up to his weight gain. To maintain a healthful weight at his height, Joe's recommended calorie allotment was around two thousand calories per day. Yet his food diary represented an intake of about sixteen hundred calories. He should have been losing weight on his low-calorie, low-fat, vegetarian diet.

Vegetarians born with Metabolism A can lose weight on a low-calorie lifestyle that excludes meat, poultry, fish, cheese, butter, milk, yogurt, and other dairy. All they need is a low-calorie program within their caloric allotment with their acceptable food choices. They will lose weight.

But that's not true for vegetarians born with Metabolism B. They are often perplexed by the fact that although they purposely modified their lifestyle to avoid meat (plus eggs and dairy, in the case of vegans) and assume that a vegetarian lifestyle will promote healthy weight and improved health, they find the exact opposite happening. They have

Joe's recent weight gain showed around his midsection. His father, who was overweight and diagnosed with type 2 diabetes, had the same shape. Joseph's dad was recently hospitalized for a TIA (mini-stroke) and was prescribed lifetime blood thinners, medication for hypertension, blood glucose, and a statin for his cholesterol. Joe was more than afraid he would end up like his father if he didn't do something now.

Joseph definitely had Metabolism B, and it had begun to wreak havoc with his new higher-carbohydrate, low-calorie diet. His vegetarian diet choices, although lower in calories and fat, were much higher in total carbohydrate. Grains, legumes, fruits, and many milk products are considered carbohydrates. His Metabolism B was overprocessing these foods and depositing fat around his middle and in his blood.

When Joe looked at the list of foods he could eat during Step One he didn't think he could make it through the eight weeks as a vegetarian because Step One temporarily cut back on carbohydrate grams. He was relieved to see that his protein needs could be met with eggs or egg whites, low-fat carb-controlled milk, low-fat cheese, soy products, tofu, nut butters, and protein drinks. He was also relieved that he could eat liberal amounts of many vegetables.

Within the first eight weeks Joseph landed in the middle of his pounds and inches target range. By the time he finished Step Two his lab work entered the normal zone. He has been able to maintain his vegetarian lifestyle easily throughout all three steps of the Metabolism Miracle. He lives on his maintenance plan and looks and feels great.

unwittingly replaced many proteins and fats with "healthy" carbohydrates, and of course Metabolism B wreaks havoc when carbohydrates enter the diet in large quantities at unscheduled times.

For lacto-ovo vegetarians (those who eat eggs and dairy), the solution lies in balancing the diet with high-value vegetarian proteins rather than depending solely on protein in carbohydrates. They can easily follow all the basic rules of every step of the Metabolism Miracle, enjoy their meals, and reap excellent results in which they lose weight and optimize their health.

Vegans require more planning to follow the Metabolism Miracle program. Because they rely completely on nonanimal and high-carbohydrate sources of protein and because Step One is an extremely low-carb phase, I recommend vegans spend a max of four weeks at a time in Step One and the other four weeks in Step Two to equal an eight-week block of MM.

During Step One protein needs can be met with soy milk, tofu, soy products, nut butters, and nuts while the pancreas and liver rest. For a vegan it's prudent to spend the rest of the weight-loss mode in Step Two, which will include 11- to 20-gram net carb servings of whole grains, legumes, and fruits. Vegans should live in Step Two until they reach their desirable healthy weight.

Step Two is more reasonable for vegans because it introduces whole grains like whole wheat and multigrain bread, brown rice, fruit, and legumes to the mix. If you are uncertain of how to adapt veganism to Steps One and Two of the Metabolism Miracle, you might want to schedule an appointment with a registered dietitian who can help you establish a plan week-by-week.

Sample Lacto-Ovo Vegetarian Menu for Step One

5:30 a.m. Wake up
6:00 a.m. Breakfast:
   omelet with egg whites, light shredded Cheddar, peppers, onions, and tomatoes; 1 slice of low-carb toast (5-gram Counter Carb) with whipped butter

9:00 a.m. Midmorning snack:
   part-skim string cheese and a handful of almonds

12:00 pm. Lunch:
   meatless burger (no carbs) with Lorraine Swiss cheese, sliced tomato and onion and topped with reduced-sugar ketchup and wrapped in lettuce leaves instead of bun; 1 cup of popcorn (no hydrogenated fat; 5-gram Counter Carb)

3:00 p.m. Afternoon snack:
   cottage cheese cup with tomato wedges; handful of pumpkin seed
   kernels

5:00 p.m. Exercise for one hour:
   1 peach before beginning exercise and 3 Gatorade Chews after a half-
   hour of exercise

7:30 p.m. Dinner:
   easy pizza made with one tortilla (5-gram Counter Carb), ½ cup of
   marinara sauce, shredded pizza cheese, peppers, onion, mushrooms,
   and Parmesan cheese; large garden salad with nuts, seeds, boiled
   egg, and balsamic vinaigrette

11:00 p.m. Bedtime snack:
   1 slice of toast (5-gram Counter Carb) with natural peanut butter and
   a glass of unsweetened chocolate almond milk

Step Two Lacto-Ovo Vegetarian Sample Menu

5:30 a.m.: Wake up
6:00 a.m. Breakfast:
   egg white omelet with light shredded cheese and veggies; 1 light
   multigrain English muffin (11- to 20-gram Carb Dam) with whipped
   butter
9:00 a.m. Midmorning snack:
   handful of peanuts; flavored yogurt (11- to 20-gram Carb Dam)

12 p.m. Lunch:
   grilled cheese sandwich with 2 slices of thin-sliced whole-grain
   bread (11- to 20-gram Carb Dam), sliced cheese, whipped butter, and
   tomato slices; sugar-free gelatin cup with whipped cream

3:00 p.m. Afternoon snack:
   1 cup of cantaloupe (11- to 20-gram Carb Dam)

5:00 p.m.:

Exercise for one hour (no Fueling Forward needed, as exercise does not exceed one hour)

7:00 p.m. Dinner:

Eggplant Rollatini (recipe on page 312) with soy meatballs (11- to 20-gram Carb Dam) and grated Parmesan cheese; spinach salad with feta cheese and vinaigrette

10:00 p.m. Bedtime snack:

Zucchini Muffin (recipe on page 332); 1 cup of fat-free milk (11- to 20-gram Carb Dam)

Step One Vegan Sample Menu

6:00 a.m. Wake up

7:00 a.m. Breakfast:

1 cup of unsweetened soy milk; 1 low-carb tortilla (5-gram Counter Carb) with natural peanut butter

10:00 a.m. Midmorning snack:

dip of soy cottage cheese with bell pepper strips

12:00 p.m. Lunch:

tofu burgers (each containing fewer than 5 grams net carb), topped with soy cheese, lettuce, tomato, and onion slices, on 1 slice of low-carb bread (5-gram Counter Carb); celery sticks with natural almond butter

3:00 p.m. Afternoon snack:

handful of a neutral mix of almonds, coconut flakes, sesame seeds, and sunflower kernels

5:00 p.m. Dinner:

spaghetti squash with ½ cup of marinara sauce simmered with Italian herbs and ground tofu browned in olive oil; 1 slice of low-carb garlic bread with olive oil and garlic (5-gram Counter Carb); large garden salad with balsamic vinaigrette

9:30 p.m. Bedtime snack:
1 slice of low-carb bread (5-gram Counter Carb) with natural peanut butter; 1 cup of almond milk

Step Two Vegan Sample Menu

7:00 a.m.: Wake up
7:30 a.m. Breakfast:
½ cup of cooked oatmeal (11- to 20-gram Carb Dam) with ⅓ cup of blueberries and chopped walnuts; 1 cup unsweetened soy milk

11:00 a.m. Midmorning snack:
1 apple (11- to 20-gram Carb Dam); handful of neutral nut mix, unsweetened coconut flakes, and sunflower seed kernels

2:00 p.m. Lunch:
large salad with crumbled tofu, sunflower seed kernels, veggies, nuts, ½ cup of chick peas (11- to 20-gram Carb Dam), and olive oil and vinegar dressing

5:00 p.m. Afternoon snack:
celery sticks with almond butter; 1 fresh peach (11- to 20-gram Carb Dam)

8:00 p.m. Dinner:
sliced Tofurkey™ (vegetarian tofu-based "turkey"); ½ sweet potato (11- to 20-gram Carb Dam); large portion of steamed broccoli with olive oil and garlic; salad with pumpkin seed kernels and vinaigrette

11:30 p.m. Bedtime Snack:
½ cup of cereal (15 grams net carb) with 1 cup of unsweetened almond milk and ⅓ cup of blueberries (5 grams net carb; total carb serving for the entire snack should equal an 11- to 20-gram Carb Dam)

Many people travel for work or simply enjoy dining out even when home. Using the same thoughtful choices that you put into home meals, the Metabolism Miracle program will work well in any restaurant. Fine dining, take-out, and even fast-food choices are easy on all three of the steps.

Step One: Be a bit of a purist during Step One. Order easy, single-item low-carb entrées such as chicken, fish, seafood, pork, or lean steak rather than a combination food or a choice with which you are unfamiliar. Avoid breading and unknown sauce. Ask your waiter about any ingredients if you are unsure of a food offering.

Because you don't have to count calories, portion sizes of protein choices are not an issue. You can also indulge at the salad bar, enjoying double portions of grilled veggies, lettuce, peppers, shredded cheese, eggs, olives, sunflower kernels, and broccoli. Just stay away from higher-carb choices such as chickpeas, croutons, beets, kidney beans, fruit salad, pasta salad, or three-bean or potato salad.

Steps Two and Three: It is even easier to eat out once you graduate to Steps Two and Three. You will be able to include breading, sauce, and hidden cornstarch, counting them as 11- to 20-gram Carb Dams. Just about any food can be worked into your recommended carb range when you are following the maintenance phase, Step Three, of the Metabolism Miracle. Save up your carb servings for dinner out, having a minimum of one carb serving at prior meals and appropriate snacks.

Twelve Tips for Eating Out, MM Style

1. *Check your watch.* Consider the number of hours between your last meal or snack and when your food will arrive at your table. If it will be close to or over the five-hour mark, remember to eat an appropriate 11- to 20-gram Carb Dam to "dam" the liver from releasing excess sugar before you even get the chance to order.

2. *Have it your way.* Don't be timid about making reasonable requests, such as dressing on the side, an extra order of vegetables to replace the potato or rice, or chicken breast without added sauce. Keep in mind that

many people have dietary considerations, and restaurants often fill special requests.

3. *Skip the bread.* Request that no bread or chip basket be brought to the table or move the basket out of sight so it stays out of mind.

4. *Order simply.* Select unbreaded meat, fish, or poultry with vegetables and salad. Skip sauces, breading, and gravies.

5. *Make salad considerations.* Avoid croutons in salads, as they contain unnecessary carbs.

6. *Replace starch with extra veggies.* Replace potato, rice, or pasta with a substitution order of healthy vegetables.

7. *Find the carb-friendly menu section.* Many restaurants accommodate dieters with low-carb sections on their menus.

8. *Check Nutrition Facts.* More and more restaurants now include Nutrition Facts on their menus. Rather than looking at their total carb grams minus net carb grams, you need to look at the contents of the meal and make sure it is all neutral veggies or neutral foods with lean, unbreaded protein and no sauce. Restaurants count every single ingredient's carbs (like carb grams in lettuce, tomato, bell peppers, cheese), so a chef's salad that would be a 5-gram carb (as we don't know exactly what is in their dressing) might show net carb grams of 18 or more when they add up all the carb grams, even in our neutral foods.

9. *Opt for meal salads.* A large salad with protein makes a great low-carb entrée. Choose chef's salad, antipasto, Cobb salad, or chicken Caesar salad without croutons.

10. *Request a sandwich sans bread.* Ask the waiter to hold the bread and to put the insides of your favorite sandwich on top of a bed of salad greens with dressing on the side.

11. *Enjoy a burger with the fixings.* Enjoy the beef, cheese, lettuce, tomato, onion, and pickle without a bun—or bring your own neutral bun!

12. *Have breakfast for lunch.* Have a western omelet (egg whites or egg substitute preferred) with cheese, vegetables, and Canadian bacon.

Chinese Take-Out

Chinese food can be full of great vegetables and fresh ingredients, but rice, noodles, sauces, and hidden thickeners make most Chinese dishes high in carbohydrate. During Step One skip the rice, noodles, fried noodles, wontons, breading, and even sauces, as most sauces include carb-heavy cornstarch.

Think about hidden carbs when you make an order. Chicken and broccoli without the rice seems like a perfect choice to order for Step One, but the sauce often contains cornstarch. It's a fine choice for Steps Two and Three when you count the sauce as an 11- to 20-gram Carb Dam. Order Chinese food with no sugar or starch when possible.

Chinese Food to Avoid on Step One
  breaded or coated meats (e.g., General Tso's chicken)
  deep-fried items
  egg rolls' crispy covering
  noodles (pasta, wontons, wrappers)
  rice (white rice, fried rice, steamed rice, rice balls)
  sweet sauces (duck/plum sauce, sweet-and-sour sauce, oyster sauce, hoisin sauce)

Chinese Food to Enjoy
  egg foo yong (without gravy)
  egg rolls' insides (don't eat the wrappers)
  Mongolian barbecue (often present at Chinese buffets; choose your own meats and veggies and request no sauce)
  mu shu without the wrappers
  soups, including egg-drop soup (count as a 5-gram Counter Carb for thickener), chicken broth with neutral veggies (count as a 5-gram Counter Carb for thickener), and hot and sour soup
  soy sauce (neutral on MM, but it is high in sodium!)
  steamed foods without sauces (order egg-drop or chicken broth on the side and use the soup as the 5-gram Counter Carb sauce for a steamed dish)
  stir-fried dishes without sugar or starch

Italian Food

Mention Italian food, and most people envision pasta, pizza, and crusty Italian bread. But native Italians don't overload with carbs as most Americans think they do. I remember searching for a slice of pizza in Rome. What I found had paper-thin crust, very light fresh tomato sauce, and a very, very small amount of cheese—nothing like the thick-crusted and greasy concoction we call pizza in the United States.

Eat like a true Italian: order fish, seafood, poultry, or meat with lots of fresh vegetables on the side. Salad is also plentiful. You can also have a glass of wine (neutral) with dinner. On Steps Two or Three you can have a small serving of pasta on the side.

Italian Food to Avoid

Lasagna with garlic bread can spell disaster for someone with Metabolism B. When I really want carb-heavy Italian food, I wait until Step Two. On Step Two I have one "off" meal per week. For that one off-meal I always choose Italian, Mexican, or Chinese food. Then back on plan I go.

Italian Food to Enjoy

Antipasti. A typical antipasti platter (the term means "before the meal") contains an assortment of meats, cheeses, marinated veggies, and olives, all acceptable in any step of the Metabolism Miracle. Other good appetizers include grilled, roasted, or marinated veggies, steamed clams or mussels, fresh mozzarella with tomatoes and basil, and shrimp sautéed in garlic and wine.

Pizza. If you crave pizza during Step One, satisfy that urge by enjoying the toppings—cheese, onions, peppers, spinach, and broccoli—and leaving the crust behind. You can also buy or make neutral pizza crust (visit www.Miracle-Ville.com to learn more).

Salads. Most contain dark greens, olive oil, and crushed garlic. Feel free to add cheese and tomatoes, but skip the croutons.

Seafood. Seafood is always a great choice, as are chicken and veal entrées with sauce on the side for flavor. Just choose options without breading and count a dip or two of sauce as your 5-gram Counter Carb.

Soups. Enjoy chicken broth with spinach, simple vegetable soup, Italian wedding soup without pasta, or Italian egg-drop soup.

Mexican Food

With its rice, beans, corn, tortillas, tacos, burritos, enchiladas, and tamales, Mexican food is steeped in carbohydrate. But there are plenty of Metabolism B–friendly choices to make in any Mexican restaurant. The trick is to count your carb servings and think about what's inside all of those tacos, tortillas, and other wraps.

One carb serving of 11 to 20 grams equals:

12 tortilla chips

½ cup of beans

½ cup of rice

2 hard taco shells

1 soft taco shell

Mexican Food to Avoid

Hold the rice and tortilla chips. Remember that while you are on Step One, you'll need to request "no rice" and shun the basket of tortilla chips. During Steps Two and Three about twelve tortilla chips, a half-cup of beans, or a half-cup of rice equals one carb serving.

Wraps, tortillas, and more. Most carbs in Mexican food come from tortilla shells, wraps, rice, and beans. Peek inside burritos, chimichangas, enchiladas, tacos, tortillas, and the like to see if what's inside will work for you: seasoned taco meat, shredded cheese, lettuce, tomato, salsa, and sour cream are all fine, even during Step One. Just remove the wrap and eat the inside.

Mexican Food to Enjoy

Ensalada. A salad is a great appetizer choice. Skip the hard tortilla shell of the tostada salad—everything inside is great.

Fajitas. Even people in Step One can enjoy all of the fajita accompaniments (shrimp, steak, chicken, guacamole, cheese, salsa, sour cream, tomato, lettuce, and onion), but skip the soft tortilla shells. One small hard taco shell equals a 5-gram Counter Carb, and eat the remainder of the hard tacos' fillings—but only one hard shell.

Grilled proteins and vegetables. Grilled seafood with a light salsa, carne asada (grilled steak with Mexican spices), and chicken dishes with grilled vegetables and salsas make very friendly fare for anyone with Metabolism B.

Guacamole and cucumber chips. Avocado is a heart-healthy fat and is fine during all steps of the Metabolism Miracle. Use cucumber slices for dipping or eat it by the spoonful!

Machaca. This common breakfast of eggs, beef, and vegetables works for Steps One, Two, and Three.

Fast Food

Fast food is always a questionable choice for anyone trying to eat healthy. But you can make decent choices when you're following the Metabolism Miracle and you find yourself at a fast-food restaurant. Also, you can check out any fast food chain's Nutrition Facts online!

Fast Food to Avoid

Skip breaded chicken and fish. Although both are lean proteins, chicken and fish when coated with a breading and then deep fried take on extra carbs and fat.

Skip fries, tots, onion rings, desserts, and shakes, which have astronomical amounts of carb, fat, and calories.

Fast Food to Enjoy

Grilled burgers. Top a grilled burger with cheese and plenty of lettuce, tomato, onions, and pickles. *Skip the bun.*

Grilled chicken. Along with cheese, lettuce, and tomato, grilled chicken makes a great meal.

McMuffin (without the English muffin). Order breakfast egg sandwiches without the bread, or remove it when you open the wrapper. Use your own 5-gram low-carb tortilla!

Salads. Many fast-food restaurants now offer salads that feature protein, such as chicken or steak, cheese, and eggs. Opt for low-fat dressing or vinaigrette. (If the dressing has a packet with Nutrition Facts, make sure two tablespoons of dressing has 3 or fewer grams of sugar. Then you can use it lightly as a neutral dressing.)

Sub sandwiches, sans bun. Skip the roll and turn the interior of a submarine sandwich—the ham, cheese, turkey, roast beef, lettuce, tomato, oil, and vinegar—into a great salad. Or bring your own low-carb bread or low-carb tortilla shell as a 5-gram Counter Carb.

Tacos. The inside of tacos works well as a meal, but toss out the shell.

At-a-Glance Shopping List for Step One

Asterisked items (*) represent 5-gram Counter Carbs—check the Nutrition Facts label to make sure they don't exceed 5 grams of net carbs.

Beverages: sugar-free flavored water; sugar-free iced tea mix; sugar-free soda sweetened with Splenda, erythritol, or stevia; sugar-free hot cocoa mix; club soda; flavored seltzer; coffee; tea; bottled water

Bread: low-carb bread*, low-carb tortilla* (5 or fewer grams net carb)

Broth or bouillon

Butter: whipped butter, butter, butter blends (combination of butter and nonhydrogenated oil)

Cheese: reduced-fat string cheese, part-skim string cheese, part-skim ricotta cheese, part-skim mozzarella cheese, 2% reduced-fat Cheddar cheese, 2% American cheese, Lorraine Swiss cheese, low-fat cheese wedges and spreadable cheese, grated Parmesan cheese, 1 to 2% cottage cheese, any low-fat cheese; *no* fat-free cheese—purchase regular cheese and just use less of it

Condiments: low-carb* or sugar-free* ketchup, mustard, dill pickles

Cooking oil spray

Cream cheese: whipped or reduced-fat

Creamer: low-fat half-and-half, regular half-and-half, light cream

Eggs: organic eggs, egg whites, egg substitutes such as Egg Beaters™

Fish: any fish or shellfish

Green tea bags

Jelly: sugar-free* (5 or fewer grams net carb) or carb-free

Lemon or lime juice

Mayonnaise: light or low-fat preferred or smaller amount of regular

Meats: lean cuts of meat such as sirloin, 85 to 93 percent ground beef, ground round, ground sirloin, flank steak, London broil, T-bone, porterhouse, rump roast

Milk:* low-carb milk (5 or fewer grams net carb)

Noodles: Konjac, Miracle, or shirataki noodles and macaroni

Nuts and peanuts: almonds, cashews, peanuts, pecans, pistachios, walnuts, or any nuts without added sugar—maximum three handfuls per day

Oils: canola, corn, olive, peanut, safflower, sunflower, vegetable

Peanut or nut butter: natural peanut butter or almond butter with no added sugar—just nuts, oil, and perhaps salt

Pork: lean cuts such as tenderloin, center-cut loin chops, Canadian bacon, ham

Poultry: skinless chicken breast, turkey breast, turkey bacon, reduced-fat turkey sausage (check Nutrition Facts for carb grams)

Protein drinks:* 1 gram net carb or less is neutral, 2 to 5 grams net carb is a 5-gram Counter Carb

Salad dressing: olive oil and balsamic vinegar, low-fat* or light* salad dressing; 3 or fewer grams sugar per two tablespoons for neutral dressing

Sour cream: light, low-fat, or a small amount of regular

Soy products: tofu, unsweetened soy milk, meat substitutes* (meat subs with 5 or fewer grams net carb per serving are neutral, so you can have more than one)

Splenda, stevia, or erythritol: packets and granulated

Supplements: multivitamin, 500 to 600 mg calcium with vitamin D, 1000 to 1200 mg of EPA and DHA combined in fish oil capsules, B-complex (B-50), vitamin D (1000 IU)

Sweets: sugar-free ice pops*, sugar-free gelatin, light whipped cream, regular whipped cream, sugar-free pudding* (5 or fewer grams net carb)

Syrup:* sugar-free* (5 or fewer grams net carb) or carb-free

Vegetables: fresh or frozen artichokes, asparagus, bean sprouts, broccoli, Brussels sprouts, cabbage, cauliflower, celery, chard, collards, cucumber, eggplant, endive, green beans, kale, lettuce, mushrooms, onions, peppers, spaghetti squash, spinach, summer squash, tomatoes, zucchini; ½ cup of the following veggies is considered to be neutral: beets, carrots, marinara sauce with no added sugar, tomato juice, tomatoes, V8™ vegetable juice

Yogurt: low-carb yogurt* (5 or fewer grams net carb)

PART THREE

Exploring Health and Life Issues

12

The Diabetes Connection

A family history of prediabetes or type 2 diabetes holds a strong link to Metabolism B. If you or a close relative has had or currently has any of the following conditions, you are on the road to type 2 diabetes. If you have metabolic syndrome, prediabetes, type 2 diabetes, hypoglycemia, or gestational diabetes, MM is the program for you.

____ Low blood sugar (hypoglycemia)

____ Gestational diabetes (diabetes related to pregnancy)

____ Prediabetes (borderline diabetes)

____ Type 2 diabetes (adult-onset diabetes)

Type 1.5 Diabetes, or LADA

Most people have heard of gestational diabetes, type 1 diabetes, and type 2 diabetes.

Over the past forty years we've seen these solid lines of delineation become blurred with the discovery of what has been called type 1.5 diabetes, or *latent autoimmune diabetes of adults* (LADA). Discovered in the 1970s and more regularly discussed since the early 1990s, many diabetes practitioners subscribe to its existence, although there is not yet a classification for LADA. Although LADA is typically diagnosed in adulthood as type 2 diabetes, within three to twelve years of the diagnosis this type of diabetes begins to look more like type 1 diabetes.

LADA accounts for roughly 10 percent of people with diabetes. It is estimated that 20 percent of those initially diagnosed as having type 2

A BLOOD SUGAR PRIMER

Hypoglycemia or Low Blood Glucose Reaction

There are two types of hypoglycemia. The first type, which can happen to a person with Metabolism B, occurs about one and a half to two hours after eating a high-carb-containing meal and is due to the Met B's pancreas over-releasing insulin. Low blood sugar causes the person to feel dizzy, lightheaded, nauseated, shaky, irritable, panicky, and ravenously hungry for carbohydrate food. Within a few minutes of eating carbohydrate, the symptoms subside. People with hypoglycemia often carry food with them "in case of emergencies" and declare to their friends, "We need to eat, now!"

Sudden mood swings and irritability often cue their friends that they mean business. This type of hypoglycemia is considered a precursor to prediabetes and type 2 diabetes.

The other type of hypoglycemia is medication induced. It occurs when a person with diabetes who takes oral medication and/or uses insulin to lower blood sugar experiences blood sugar below the normal range. People on glucose-lowering medication for diabetes are strongly advised to carry glucose tablets or another source of quick-acting carbohydrate.

See page 232 for how to treat hypoglycemia.

Gestational Diabetes or Diabetes During Pregnancy

About 6 percent of pregnant women develop high blood glucose between weeks 24 and 28 of pregnancy. Diet changes, exercise, and, in some cases, insulin injections are used to keep the condition under control until delivery, when most glucose levels return to normal. Babies born to women with uncontrolled gestational diabetes often tip the scales at close to or over nine pounds. These women have a greater chance of a subsequent pregnancy with gestational diabetes and of developing type 2 diabetes in the future.

Prediabetes

Think of prediabetes as a red-flag alert. Also known as *borderline diabetes* or "a touch of sugar," this gray area between perfectly normal blood sugar and a diagnosis of type 2 diabetes offers a chance to prevent or at least slow down the progression with appropriate diet and exercise.

If you have prediabetes, you are lucky to have this opportunity to positively impact your medical future. The Metabolism Miracle is the only weight-loss program for you.

	Normal	Prediabetes	Type 2 diabetes
Fasting blood sugar (in mg/dL)	65 to 99	100 to 125	126* or greater
2 hours after eating (in mg/dL)	less than 140	greater than 140 but less than 200	200 or greater
Hemoglobin A1C	Under 5.7	5.7 to 6.4	6.5 or higher

*Type 2 diabetes should have two fasting blood glucose and/or hemoglobin A1C for diagnosis.

Type 2 Diabetes

A diagnosis of type 2 diabetes is usually made when two fasting blood glucose and/or hemoglobin A1C readings are in the type 2 diabetes zone.

Type 2 diabetes is caused by a combination of factors: a fatigued pancreas that can no longer produce adequate insulin and an increased resistance to that insulin from the very cells that need it (insulin resistance).

After years of overproducing insulin due to uncontrolled Metabolism B and prediabetes, the pancreas tires and starts to produce less and less insulin. Fat cells have increased in size, and their insulin receptors' shape has distorted in the process. As a result, cells became resistant to insulin.

The pancreas is pressured to produce more and more insulin in the hope that more insulin might find more connections. This vicious cycle permanently impairs the pancreas's ability to produce adequate insulin. At this point there is excess insulin and excess glucose in the bloodstream.

If you are overweight, inactive, and under mental or physical stress and one of your parents has type 2 diabetes, your chances of developing the disease are high. When untreated or treated incorrectly, diabetes can cause irreversible and ongoing harm, including heart disease, blindness, nerve damage, and kidney damage. The good news is that even with a genetic predisposition to type 2 diabetes, you can improve your chance to avoid this irreversible condition by losing weight, increasing physical activity, and reducing the stressors in your life. And if you already have type 2 diabetes, you can control the condition with proper diet, physical activity, blood glucose monitoring, and medicine when required.

diabetes actually have LADA. There is still uncertainty over how to define LADA and why it develops and progresses.

Often a person with LADA may be lean or normal weight when diagnosed. Oral medications may initially work to decrease elevated blood sugar. Over time (in much shorter order than in typical type 2 diabetes) oral medications become ineffective. Blood sugar worsens, and insulin must be prescribed to control high blood glucose.

Some diabetes practitioners recommend that in adult patients who present as lean or normal weight and have no known family history of type 2 diabetes, antibody testing should be performed to differentiate between type 2 diabetes and LADA.

Why would it be beneficial to "know in advance" if a person has type 2 or LADA? Well, think of it this way: many oral medications work by forcing the pancreas to produce more insulin. Sulfonylureas are one class of diabetes drugs that cause the pancreas to work harder. By prescribing more and more pancreas-provoking oral medications, to no avail, the medication would speed the demise of beta cells.

Also, if a person has LADA and is prescribed a traditional diet for diabetes (the calorie-controlled/low-fat diet), he is exposing the pancreas to high carbohydrate intake and an increased need to produce insulin caused by the high blood sugar rendered from the diet. In the same way that some oral medications press the pancreas to produce more insulin, so too does the higher carbohydrate diet require more insulin production.

In the years it takes to prove that oral medications are not working, the patient is subjected to higher than necessary hemoglobin A1C. The

FIRST THINGS FIRST

Before beginning any diet or exercise program, contact your physician. This is particularly important if you have diabetes and are taking oral medication or insulin to control blood sugar. The Metabolism Miracle will help you to lose weight and decrease blood sugar, blood pressure, and blood lipids, and those changes may warrant a change in your medication or dosage.

Keep your doctor abreast of weight losses of ten pounds or more and always report symptoms that might indicate overmedication.

fastest method to control and normalize blood glucose, the better the long-term outcomes. If insulin use is inevitable and orals can actually stress a pancreas that has begun to degrade, why not remove that excess stress from the pancreas of the person with LADA?

The Metabolism Miracle is designed to control blood sugar for those with LADA.

Will Every Person with Metabolism B Develop Type 2 Diabetes?

For a long time the medical community thought type 2 diabetes, hypertension, and high cholesterol came as the direct result of an excessive intake of calories and lack of physical activity. We now know that the genetic predisposition for excess insulin release and insulin resistance starts this process for people with Metabolism B.

Everyone with Metabolism B has the *potential* to develop type 2 diabetes, but not everyone will. You cannot develop type 2 diabetes without the genetic predisposition for the disease, the same predisposition as Metabolism B. Think of diabetes as the last stop of the Metabolism B train. It appears that a combination of being born with the gene and environmental stressors moves the train through the stops of midline weight, to elevated blood pressure, to elevated lipids, to elevated blood glucose, to prediabetes, and finally to type 2 diabetes. When a person who is born with Metabolism B is exposed to certain environmental triggers (page 229), his or her chances of developing type 2 diabetes will increase.

The greater the number of environmental factors the person with Metabolism B is exposed to, the greater his or her chances of developing diabetes.

A Complication of Type 2 Diabetes and Prediabetes: Neuropathy

Neuropathy is a complication of sustained levels of high blood glucose over a long period of time. Even those with prediabetes can develop neuropathy. Common symptoms include numbness, pain, and tingling in

TREATING HYPOGLYCEMIA

If you are *not* taking medication to lower blood sugar (oral medication or insulin), you should not experience hypoglycemia on the Metabolism Miracle. If you *are* taking medication for diabetes, please inform your physician before you begin MM because after a few days on Step One you may find the amount of medication you are taking in conjunction with MM is lowering blood sugar below the normal range.

Treat any hypoglycemia immediately and then inform your healthcare provider. Many physicians reduce their patients' diabetes medications in half when they begin the program.

Treating Hypoglycemia Caused by Excess Diabetes Medication

Typical Diabetes Drug-Induced Hypoglycemia
If blood sugar is between 50 to 70 mg/dL (2.8 mmol/L to 3.9 mmol/L), choose *one* of the following treatments:

3 to 4 glucose tabs
3 Gatorade Chews
1 cup (8 ounces) of regular Gatorade
½ cup (4 ounces) of juice
½ can (6 ounces) of regular soda
3 packets of sugar in water
1 container of regular Jell-O (½ cup)

the legs and feet, and neuropathy can impact all the nerves of the body. The only solution is to normalize blood glucose quickly and for a prolonged period of time.

Peripheral neuropathy usually affects the feet and legs.
Symptoms include:

- tingling
- numbness (may become permanent)
- burning (especially in the evening)
- pain

continued ...

Severe Hypoglycemia

If blood sugar is less than 50 mg/dL (2.8 mmol/L), choose *one* treatment from the list below:

6 to 8 glucose tabs

6 Gatorade Chews

8 ounces regular Gatorade

1 cup (8 ounces) of regular juice

12 ounces (1 can) of regular soda

6 packets of sugar in a glass of water

2 containers (2½ cups) of regular Jell-O

After you treat the hypoglycemia, wait ten to fifteen minutes, retest, and confirm that blood sugar has risen to the 80 to 120 mg/dL range (4.4 to 6.7 mmol/L).

If blood glucose remains under 70 mg/dL (3.9 mmol/L), re-treat as above (based on what your blood glucose is after treatment number one) and test again in ten minutes. Be sure to inform your physician of your hypoglycemic reaction for a possible medication decrease. After two separate blood tests that show hypoglycemia and proper treatment, if you still are hypoglycemic, call 911.

Autonomic neuropathy usually affects the stomach, intestines, and the heart, but it can also affect the blood vessels, urinary system, and sex organs.

Symptoms include:

- bloating
- diarrhea
- constipation
- heartburn
- nausea
- vomiting
- feeling full after small meals
- erratic blood sugar despite taking diabetes medications as directed

- blacking out when you stand up quickly
- faster heartbeat
- dizziness
- low blood pressure
- trouble emptying your bladder
- incontinence (leaking urine)
- more bathroom trips at night
- in men, inability to have or keep an erection and reduced ejaculation
- in women, decreased vaginal lubrication and fewer or no orgasms

The number-one way to prevent or treat neuropathy is long-term tight control of blood glucose, proper diet and lifestyle, and medication if needed to normalize blood glucose.

If you are diagnosed with peripheral or autonomic neuropathy, a long-term lifetime lifestyle that quickly and permanently controls blood glucose is the Metabolism Miracle.

13

What You Should Know About Weight-Loss Surgery

Weight-loss surgery has gained acceptance as a treatment for those with obesity or morbid obesity. Morbid obesity is classified as greater than one hundred pounds above ideal body weight or BMI 40 or higher with or without medical complications, or as less than one hundred pounds overweight if the patient has weight-related complications such as diabetes, hypertension, hyperlipidemia (cholesterol/triglycerides), blood pressure, atherosclerosis, vascular disease, and so forth. There are four common types of weight-loss surgery: Roux-en-Y gastric bypass, or gastric bypass; laparoscopic adjustable gastric banding, also called "the band"; sleeve gastrectomy, known as the "sleeve"; and duodenal switch with biliopancreatic diversion.

Roux-en-Y Gastric Bypass: Gastric Bypass

This is the full name of the most common type of gastric bypass. During this procedure the surgeon creates a very small, golf-ball-sized pouch at the top of the stomach that limits the food and drink that can be ingested at one time. A typical stomach capacity is about fifty ounces; the initial size of the stomach pouch is only about two ounces. The pouch is separated from the main stomach by staples.

In the second part of the gastric bypass the small intestine is cut a short distance below the stomach. The short end of the now-shortened small intestine is attached to the small stomach pouch so food and beverages will move from the mouth to the esophagus to the stomach pouch to the shortened small intestine; the portion of the intestine still attached to the main stomach is reattached farther down. This allows the digestive juices to flow to the small intestine. Because food now *bypasses* a portion of the small intestine, fewer nutrients and calories are absorbed.

Laparoscopic Adjustable Gastric Banding: The Band

A band containing a balloon is placed around the upper part of stomach, creating a "stomach pouch." This pouch fills quickly and, due to the small opening to the rest of the stomach, keeps the patient feeling full for a longer time. The band is removable and can be adjusted tighter or looser by utilizing saline injections in a port placed under the skin of the abdomen.

A gastric band aids in weight loss by restricting the amount of food consumed at one time. Fluids freely pass through the band, so many people find that drinking shakes, ice cream, pudding, cream soups, smoothies, and yogurt will move easier through the banded stomach; meat and veggies can cause pain and a feeling of being overly full. The weight-loss results after a band is placed are much less than those from gastric bypass, sleeve gastrectomy, or switch surgery, but the band is removable and does not restructure your GI anatomy.

Sleeve Gastrectomy: The Sleeve

In a sleeve gastrectomy part of the stomach is separated and removed from the body. The remaining section of the stomach is formed into a tube-like structure. This smaller stomach pouch cannot hold as much food and also produces less of the appetite-regulating hormone ghrelin, which may lessen the desire to eat. However, sleeve gastrectomy does not affect the absorption of calories and nutrients in the intestine.

Duodenal Switch with Biliopancreatic Diversion

As with sleeve gastrectomy, this procedure begins with the surgeon removing a large part of the stomach. The valve that releases food to the small intestine is left, along with the first part of the small intestine, called the duodenum.

The difference? The surgeon surgically closes off the *middle* section of the small intestine (the jejunum) and attaches the last part (ileum) directly to the duodenum. The jejunum is reattached to the end of the small intestine, allowing bile and pancreatic digestive juices to flow into this part of the intestine. This is the biliopancreatic diversion.

As a result of these changes, food bypasses most of the small intestine, limiting the absorption of calories and nutrients. This, together with the smaller size of the stomach, leads to weight loss.

When the weight loss stops, however, weight regain typically restarts. About a year and a half to three years after this weight-loss surgery, the two-ounce stomach pouch has stretched in size to accommodate approximately eight ounces.

At about the two-year mark after weight-loss surgery, those with Metabolism B usually note that their weight loss has slowed down and, over time, eventually stops. Unfortunately, after succeeding to lose a large amount of weight during the first year or two, they will eventually begin to regain weight. This is not a failed surgery—this is Met B becoming uncontrolled.

Although the surgery bypasses the duodenum of the small intestine, it does not bypass the genes for Metabolism B. Ironically, many of these patients end up needing to follow the Metabolism Miracle after having permanently rewired their GI tract.

The only weight-loss procedure that does not cut the stomach and/or reconstruct the small intestine's connection to the stomach is the gastric band. The success rate for this procedure is much less than bypass, and many gastric band patients eventually undergo gastric bypass.

In my practice 80 percent of patients who sought counseling for pre- or postgastric bypass had uncontrolled Metabolism B. I would advise them to follow the program for four months to see whether they were able to lose significant weight and keep it off without major surgery. Almost every patient declined to try the MM program before surgery; they moved right on to the surgery. And almost every patient required MM a few years after their surgery, even though their digestive tract was permanently reconstructed.

14

Breast Cancer and Met B

The numbers don't lie: breast cancer is an epidemic. Consider these statistics:

- One in eight women in the United States will develop invasive breast cancer during their lifetime.
- Close to two thousand cases of invasive breast cancer were expected to be diagnosed in men in 2010.
- About 70 to 80 percent of breast cancers occur in women who have no family history of breast cancer.

Obesity has long been recognized as a breast cancer risk factor. Researchers have also acknowledged the link between higher-than-normal levels of estrogen and breast cancer. As it turns out, overweight or obese women have higher estrogen levels than their normal-weight counterparts, and they also have a higher risk of breast cancer.

The majority of overweight or obese women also produce excess amounts of another hormone, the fat-gain hormone, insulin.

One study, published in the *Journal of the National Cancer Institute*, showed the link between high insulin levels and the risk of breast cancer even in the face of controlled estrogen levels.[1] The majority of breast cancer cases occur in postmenopausal women. Excess insulin production places postmenopausal women at an increased risk for breast cancer.

In the same way the largest study of postmenopausal women by the National Institutes of Health, the Women's Health Initiative, concluded that women with the highest insulin levels were twice as likely to develop breast cancer compared with women with the lower insulin levels.[2]

According to research, the hormonal imbalance of insulin may be increasing the risk for developing breast cancer, and this imbalance may also decrease the effectiveness of breast cancer treatment. Furthermore, patients with diabetes have a higher risk of developing several types of cancer, including cancer of the breast, liver, pancreas, colon, and ovaries.[3]

Overweight or obese women with high insulin levels—those who are not yet diagnosed with diabetes—are also at high risk for breast cancer. Even lean women with high insulin levels are more susceptible to breast cancer than they would be if their insulin levels were normal. Thus, considering the possible risks for developing breast cancer, especially for postmenopausal women, excess insulin is an issue that should be normalized and monitored closely.

A Simple Screening Insulin Test for
All Postmenopausal Women May Save Lives

Dr. Howard Strickler, senior author of the Einstein College study, stated, "It is also possible that screening non-diabetic postmenopausal women for high insulin levels could prove useful in identifying individuals at high risk for breast cancer."

Screening all postmenopausal women for fasting insulin levels makes sense. During these checkups fasting insulin should be 8 or less. If there is elevation, the woman needs to work to normalize insulin through effective diet, physical activity, and insulin-lowering medications such as metformin (see page 142–143).

15

Insulin and Alzheimer's Disease (AD)

Two Causes of Dementia:
Alzheimer's Disease and Vascular Dementia

Vascular dementia affects about 25 percent of those with dementia and gradually damages blood vessels that deliver nutrients to the brain. Diabetes and dementia have long been linked.

Of those with dementia, 60 to 80 percent have Alzheimer's disease (AD). Alzheimer's disease is fatal and marked by progressive loss of memory and cognition. It is characterized by abnormal protein plaques in the brain.

Both vascular dementia and Alzheimer's are defined as loss of brain function that affects a person's memory, thinking, language, judgment, and behavior.

AD now affects 15 million people worldwide. With the rapid aging of the population, upward of 14 million Americans are projected to develop Alzheimer's in the coming decades.

Experts estimate that at this time one in eight Americans ages sixty-five and over has AD, and nearly half of Americans have the disease once they reach age eighty-five.

Major research studies now link diabetes to Alzheimer's disease. The precise link between diabetes and AD is not yet known, but studies indicate that those with prediabetes and type 2 diabetes are at higher risk for developing AD.

Because the brain does not require insulin to fuel its cells, it had long been assumed that the brain was an insulin-independent organ. We are now learning that insulin may have a very different job in the brain, as the "right amount of insulin" in the brain may actually prevent Alzheimer's disease.

Insulin plays a key role in learning and memory and in the process of creating memories. A normal level of insulin going to the brain prevents proteins from gumming up and forming plaques that cause the connections between nerves to fail.

The presence of insulin in the brain enables signaling between nerves, helping messages and memories to pass from nerve to nerve. If adequate amounts of insulin are not available for "insulin signaling," learning and memory are compromised, and this may lead to Alzheimer's disease.

In the case of metabolic syndrome, prediabetes, type 2 diabetes, and long-term and worsening type 2 diabetes, insulin imbalance causes difficulty with messages and memories passing between nerves. As prediabetes and type 2 diabetes progress, so does insulin resistance and the eventual decrease of insulin production. As insulin resistance worsens, the pancreas gradually fatigues, and the amount of insulin to the brain decreases. Low insulin to the brain causes sticky amyloid protein to build and gum up the connections between the nerves as well as form plaques in the brain. As insulin resistance worsens, there is a marked breakdown of nerve connections in the brain.

Alzheimer's involves the nervous and the endocrine system, and for this reason, it is sometimes referred to as "type 3 diabetes" (type 1 and type 2 diabetes also involve nerves and the endocrine system). Those with type 2 diabetes have an increased risk of heart attack, stroke, and Alzheimer's disease. Diabetes is a risk factor for ALL forms of dementia. Thus, taking steps to prevent or control type 2 diabetes—to control Metabolism B—may actually help reduce the risk of AD.

16

High Cholesterol and Statins

Cholesterol is needed to build cells and make hormones. A healthy body is able to make all the cholesterol it needs; cholesterol is made in the liver. When we overeat foods that are high in dietary cholesterol, the natural cholesterol balance becomes unbalanced, and hyperlipidemia (high cholesterol and triglycerides) can develop.

Medications known as statins block the production of a substance your liver needs to make cholesterol, and they might also help your body reabsorb cholesterol that has already accumulated in your arteries. Statins may do more than just lower cholesterol, however; they also appear to be anti-inflammatory, which could affect many areas of the body beyond the heart. Statins began being prescribed in 1987, and today many adults (and some children) have been prescribed statins to lower their cholesterol. Well-known statins include atorvastatin (Lipitor™), fluvastatin (Lescol™), rosuvastatin (Crestor™), and simvastatin (Zocor™). Usually the decision to start a statin is based upon a few numbers on your lab work, LDL over 130 and total cholesterol over 199, but the numbers alone aren't the deciding factor. Whether you would benefit from being on a statin also depends on other risk factors for heart disease.

The general recommendation for total cholesterol is 200 mg/dL or less. LDL cholesterol (bad cholesterol) should be under 100 mg/dL, and for those at high cardiac risk, statins will help keep LDL cholesterol at or under 70 mg/dL.

In addition to your cholesterol numbers, your level of risk also includes your age, race, gender, blood pressure, and whether you have diabetes or smoke.

The American College of Cardiology and American Heart Association issued guidelines on the four main factors that would indicate statins:[1]

- *If you have cardiovascular disease,* including heart attacks, strokes, peripheral artery disease, or have had surgery to open or replace coronary arteries.
- *If you have very high LDL (bad) cholesterol,* at levels of 190 mg/dL (4.9 mmol/L) or higher.
- *If you have diabetes* and an LDL between 70 and 189 mg/dL (1.8 and 4.9 mmol/L), especially if you have evidence of vascular disease.
- *If you have a higher ten-year risk of heart attack,* meaning you have an LDL above 100 mg/dL (1.8 mmol/L) and your ten-year risk of a heart attack is 7.5 percent or higher.

The potential side effects of statins include muscle pain, liver and/or kidney damage, increased blood sugar or progression to type 2 diabetes, memory loss, headache, and nausea. Especially if you have liver or kidney disease or other health problems, it's important to consider these and other side effects before you start taking statins. You should also speak with your doctor about whether statins interact with other drugs or supplements you might be taking.

Taking statins is usually a lifetime commitment. If your LDL cholesterol level decreases after you take a statin, you'll likely stay on it indefinitely. Cholesterol levels often go back up if you remove the statin.

The exception may be if you lose weight or make significant lifestyle changes, but don't change your medications without talking to your doctor first. Following the Metabolism Miracle program could be the proper diet, exercise, and lifestyle to help markedly lower your LDL cholesterol.

17

Stories from the Field

One of the truths about Metabolism B is that it affects so many different people of many different ages from many different walks of life. I've seen thousands of patients over the past thirty-five years, and since the development of this program I've watched a lot of transformations take place as the Metabolism Miracle works its magic. The following stories represent just a few of the many different people who have benefited from the program and moved from despair to empowerment.

Caitlin Lost 110 Pounds and Traded a Size 22 for a Size 6

Caitlin regained health, energy, and confidence with the Metabolism Miracle. This is her story.

I was diagnosed with PCOS after my husband and I had a miscarriage in 2010. I weighed 251 pounds, and I hadn't had a cycle for two years. It was a miracle that my husband and I were able to conceive in the first place. We lost the baby in October.

After this sad time in my life, I decided I would no longer give in to my food addiction and would start "getting healthy." I'm young, and I wanted to live a healthy, unencumbered life.

I chose a new OB/Gyn and made an appointment with an endocrinologist for my PCOS. The endocrinologist prescribed diet pills. For those who don't know, diet pills are "speed." They artificially ramp up your heart rate and cause weight loss because you are always "running" without a break. Diet pills are very hard on the heart, cause anxiety, take away sleep, and are addictive. Once you stop them—and you will have to stop taking them—you gain back more weight than you lost.

I stopped taking diet pills because of the cost and health effects. After stopping the drugs, I stuck to a twelve-hundred-calorie-a-day diet and really worked out. I actually ended up gaining eighteen pounds in one month.

I realized that something was very wrong. A low-calorie diet *and* exercise should result in weight loss, not gain. I was so frustrated and upset. I didn't know where to turn.

My dad sent me *The Metabolism Miracle.* As I read it, everything in that book sounded like it was written for me. My father has type 2 diabetes and already had great success with this program and no longer requires medication for diabetes.

I literally started the program the next day. I have lost over 110 pounds and traded in my size 22 for a size 6, and I am still losing weight.

I want to inspire others to do this program. Those with PCOS, metabolic syndrome, prediabetes, and type 2 diabetes can't lose weight and get healthy by decreasing calories and exercising because those with these endocrinologic conditions have a different type of metabolism.

Since following the Metabolism Miracle my adult acne has cleared up, my emotions and moods are *a lot* more even, I no longer crave sugar, I have so much self-confidence, and I feel more like myself than I ever have before.

Losing weight is difficult—if it were easy, everybody would do it. But with the Metabolism Miracle you can do it.

Best wishes, Caitlin

Ava, Thirty-Two Years Old and Considering Gastric Bypass Surgery

A businesswoman appeared at my office to fulfill the surgeon's requirement that she meet with a registered dietitian before she could be scheduled for gastric bypass surgery.

Ava and I began to talk, and she related that she was mad about being forced to meet with yet another dietitian. She had worked with RDs before and never had success. All she wanted was her surgery so she could go on to live a leaner and more productive life. She was sure her weight was getting in the way of promotions at work.

At thirty-two years of age, Ava was five-foot-four and weighed 220 pounds. She explained that until her early twenties she was a much smaller version of her present self. She ran five days a week and followed a low-calorie diet. She managed to maintain a weight of 120 pounds and had energy, self-esteem, and motivation to enter the business world.

When Ava was twenty-three her mother passed away from breast cancer. Her mom had always struggled with her weight and took medications for cholesterol and high blood pressure. Toward the end of her life, Ava's mom was told she had "flipped over" to type 2 diabetes.

After dealing with her beloved mom's illness and death, Ava stopped exercising, relied on fast food, gave in to her many food cravings, and felt depressed and miserable. The pounds packed on. Nine years later she had gained a hundred pounds. Her clothes didn't fit right and she was anxious, had a new case of adult acne, fell asleep at two major meetings, and was not finishing her reports on time.

I assessed Ava's personal symptoms. She carried a good portion of her weight around her middle. She complained about being depressed and about the way she looked and felt. She recently suffered a panic attack on the train into the city. She described herself as a carb addict, craving salty and crunchy snack foods as well as chocolate, and she couldn't seem to stop eating because she never really felt full. She recently began to drink coffee for energy, but she reported no pick-me-up from the added caffeine.

Ava's fasting lab data showed a high blood glucose level, high LDL and low HDL cholesterol, and a low level of vitamin D.

It was clear to me, given her weight gain, midline fat deposits, family history of diabetes, personal symptoms, and present lab work that she had Metabolism B and could benefit hugely from the Metabolism Miracle. Ava, however, had come to my office to get the "I met with the dietitian box" checked off on her presurgery questionnaire.

I told Ava that gastric bypass is a permanent rearrangement of the GI tract but that the procedure does not bypass the genes for Metabolism B. She might lose a hundred or more pounds in a little more or less than a year, but when her stomach stretched to a certain capacity, about eight ounces, her carb cravings and intake would trip up her pancreas's hyperactivity and cause weight gain again.

I asked Ava to consider giving my program a four-month chance. If at the end of four months she still wanted to go through with the surgery, I would understand. She decided to give the Metabolism Miracle a chance with the understanding that if it didn't work for her, I would check the dietitian box to clear her for surgery. I planned to see her at eight weeks to check her progress. I recorded her starting weight and body measurements and entered them into her chart.

At eight weeks a new Ava appeared, looking bright, healthy, happy, and confident. She had lost twenty-one pounds of fat tissue, which gives the appearance of thirty-one to thirty-six pounds of weight loss on traditional diets. Her inches lost and pounds lost matched each other. Her new lab data was markedly improved, with glucose and cholesterol in the normal range. She was exercising by briskly walking forty-five minutes five times a week. She did Fuel Forward. Her clothes were loose, and she mentioned that she was hooking her bra two links smaller! She had energy, felt peaceful, and was hopeful.

She was hesitant about adding the required carbohydrate grams for Step Two because in the past, when she reintroduced carbohydrate in Phase Two of another popular low-carb diet, she regained all of her weight. Taking a leap of faith, however, Ava moved on to Step Two and returned in two months after losing fifteen additional pounds of fat and fourteen inches. Her total weight loss during the sixteen-week period was thirty-six pounds, which looks like forty-six to fifty-one pounds on a traditional diet.

I asked Ava what she had decided about the surgery after four months on MM. She smiled and said, "I think I can take it from here. I am doing an excellent job, feel great, look great, and know I can do this as a lifestyle." And she did.

Chris Lost 230 Pounds, 32 Inches Off His Waist, 7 Shirt Sizes, 5 Shoe Widths, and 10 Inches Off His Neck

Chris did all of this while he regained his health, wellness, and life! The Metabolism Miracle *is* a miracle! This is his story.

February 1, 2012, was a good day. Maybe the best of days. Oh, I'm certain I didn't feel that way at the time, but sometimes things aren't what they seem. I'm guessing I was pretty scared that day. I know I have been that and much more many days since. Just a few days prior I knew who I was, what I was doing, and where I was going.

I feel much the same way four years later, but I don't recognize the guy in the photos from back then. That is to say, while I recognize the photo, I have no recognition of who he was, what he was doing, or where he was going. While the physical changes are undeniable, the thought processes are all profoundly different. I suppose they must be.

I can recite a bunch of measurements to tell you how much I've physically changed, things like 32 inches in the waist, 10 inches in the neck, 7 shirt sizes, 5 shoe widths, and 230 pounds—all lost. What I can't quantify in mathematical terms are the things I have gained. I suppose I could say I've gained my life. That ought to express the magnitude of the gains. Or I've gained confidence, peace, wisdom, knowledge, perspective, or a dozen others. Pick a noun of profound importance. Here's the rub: I never want to go back to that panicked, nervous, sick, near-sighted, carb-addicted life I had. Why? Because I've never felt better or more free. Not only because I can move, but more importantly because I have peace. The world sees that the fat guy gets thin, but that is no more than a very tiny tip of a really big iceberg. The internal emotions and thoughts have changed more than I could've imagined. I've been blessed over the last four years to be sure. Forty more? Well, one never knows.

I get asked a lot how I've done what I've done—several times after my latest post marking the four-year anniversary of my start date. While I found it easy, or at least that is my recollection, I can say that it is more complicated than I can post at once. Mainly because it's been four years of work, and I have changed/modified things along the way. You see, a plan gets one started, but then learning one's triggers and tolerances, listening to one's body, noticing small changes, and tweaking the lifestyle is complicated and very important. Most folks are just looking to get started, so let me give some five-thousand-foot views to getting started.

The first plan that I used and had good success with for many reasons was the Metabolism Miracle by Diane Kress. The reason I liked it was for its simplicity. I needed easy at that point in my life. The second reason I liked it was that it works. I like things that work. Her book, *The Metabolism Miracle Cookbook,* provides a list that is easy to read and understand, recipes that are tasty, and support if needed. I lost about 150 pounds in eighteen months following her plan. The third thing I liked about her is that she lived this. This isn't some corporate entity shipping you a box of goo because a former athlete tells you it works. This is a professional who walks the walk and talks the talk. Diane's story told me she knew where I was and, more importantly, where I needed to go.

I could go on and on some more about Diane, the Metabolism Miracle, and the Diabetes Miracle, but it is the reason I've lost the weight, got off the meds, and live happily today. I still use the Arrow Sheet from that book and have handed a copy of the book to many people along the way—I keep an extra copy on the shelf just for that purpose. Some have paid it forward as well. Suffice it to say, if you want to change your life, reduce the medications you take, live healthier, and lose weight, this is the way to do it.

—*Chris*

Kimberly Lost Forty-Two Pounds in Six Months and Has Now Lost a Total of Fifty Pounds After the Births of Her Four Children!

I started the Metabolism Miracle in May of 2014 when I was at 251 pounds. I am now at 199 pounds! I am finally losing the weight and becoming healthier, and I couldn't be more thrilled. I still have more to lose, but for the first time in over a decade I now believe I will do it.

I was always really thin as a child and young adult. After the birth of my first child I was able to lose all the baby weight by following Weight Watchers™. After the birth of my second child something was different. The weight would not come off like before. I was able to lose twenty or so pounds, but I couldn't progress any further. And then I regained the weight, plus more!

I then had babies number three and four. And the weight just kept piling on. I tried every diet out there. I had prepackaged meals, I counted calories, I exercised, and I even tried diet pills. I was desperate to lose the weight. I knew something must be wrong with my body, but nothing concrete would show up in my lab work.

I did notice that my fasting glucose was creeping up. (It used to be very low.) And my cholesterol was now borderline high. I was then diagnosed with polycystic ovary syndrome (PCOS).

The doctors would tell me to lose weight. I knew they didn't believe me when I said I was following diets very strictly. It was very frustrating. I felt like a failure. After finding *The Metabolism Miracle* my life has changed. I have lost over fifty pounds, and I feel great.

This lifestyle has changed my life. My cholesterol is now perfect. My PCOS symptoms are completely managed, and, best of all, I am finally losing the weight and keeping it off!

—*Kimberly*

Brian's Story:
Down 72.5 Pounds, Looking Good, Feeling Great

I am still as pumped about MM as I was when I started, and I try to share it with anyone who will listen—and some who don't even want to listen!

I knew long ago that something seemed off with my body. During all those years I didn't even know what a metabolism was or how it applied to me. What I did know was that people all around me seemed to be able to eat whatever they wanted, as much as they wanted, and as often as they wanted and didn't have a weight issue like mine. I was watching what I ate, how much I ate, and when I ate. I was trying very hard to lose weight but could not succeed. It was so frustrating.

I admit that I *love* food and enjoy eating. So keeping portions down to tiny amounts of protein and half-cup of this, half-cup of that was *very* difficult—and without results.

I told myself, "If I have to give up my fun time to exercise myself to death, or if I have to eat like a rabbit for the rest of my life to keep weight off, I'm just not going to do it. I mean, what's the point of living if you aren't happy?" And I wasn't happy starving and sweating to the oldies.

I kept gaining weight until—wham—I was diagnosed with type 2 diabetes. I had to do something and I had to do it fast. I was about a year out from my commercial fishing license renewal so I knew I had time to get started with a program to control blood sugar, I might have enough time to save my job.

I searched the web for the right program for me. I needed a diet for diabetes.

I downloaded five books, and *The Metabolism Miracle* was among them. I kept going back to the Metabolism Miracle diet because one very important point kept jumping out at me: the Metabolism Miracle is designed to control a metabolism that can progress to type 2 diabetes. The book actually explained in a way I could understand what happened to me and how my metabolism differed.

I kept reading the book and saying, "That's exactly what's happening." Here was something I could almost touch—I could feel it because I was living what this book was explaining.

Within a short period of time on Metabolism Miracle my hemoglobin A1C dropped from 8.2 to 6.2. A few months later it dropped to 4.7. I didn't require diabetes medication. I started MM with an average blood sugar of 186 and now had an average blood sugar of 85! My body dealt with a 17-pound weight gain in the process of lowering blood sugar and I have lost a total of 55 pounds on the scale plus 17.5 pounds from decreasing my A1C by 3.5 points on the fat-burning steps of the program. Total weight loss: 72.5 pounds!

I'm currently at my target weight. My pant size dropped from a 40 waist to 33! That's seven inches off my waist alone. I'm comfortable and happy at my present weight.

I also use video games, television, or a phone call with a friend to take my mind off exercise while I'm on my recumbent bike. Before I know it, I have exceeded thirty minutes and find myself riding forty or fifty minutes—or even an hour. There are lots of mental tricks that can help you feel that exercise is not drudgery. AND THEY WORK!

P.S. I retained my commercial fishing license and still have my job!

—Brian

Beth: Upcoming Knee Surgery for
This Retired Physical Therapist

After years of procrastinating, sixty-year-old Beth, a retired physical therapist, saw the orthopedic surgeon she had worked for to set up a date for a knee replacement. She was almost embarrassed to need the surgery, as she always focused on physical therapy and felt she was taking care of business. At this point Beth felt depressed, old, stiff, and needed a cane to walk. During routine presurgery testing Beth was surprised to hear she had prediabetes, hypertension, and low vitamin D.

As Beth thought about it, the years between having a sore knee and a bone-on-bone knee really decreased her walking and physical activity. It was the reason she retired early. During that time she had gained some weight and acquired high blood pressure. But when and why did prediabetes enter her world?

Beth needed to lose weight, lower her blood pressure, and normalize her blood glucose before her surgery. She smiled when she entered my office, saying, "I need a three-fer." As a physical therapist, she knew weight loss would help her properly rehabilitate after surgery and would put less pressure on her new knee, but she honestly didn't know where to begin with her diet, as she "couldn't possibly exercise at this point."

Based on her diagnosis of prediabetes and hypertension, we decided the Metabolism Miracle matched her metabolism needs and would help her lose weight quickly and permanently. It could also prevent her progression to type 2 diabetes, and the weight loss would help lower her blood pressure.

Beth blushed when I reminded her that she didn't have to use her legs for exercise. She would continue her usual walking, but she could add exercise by using light hand weights and do muscle-toning activities in an armchair until the physical therapy after surgery. She was pleased to learn that MM wasn't about how many calories you burn but about energizing muscle tissue. She was thrilled that her physical therapy sessions would count toward her exercise time.

After completing eight weeks on Step One and eight weeks on Step Two, Beth was proud when we weighed and remeasured her, showed that she had lost thirty-two pounds and thirty-four inches. Her labs and blood pressure were cleared for surgery.

She had her double knee replacement and began physical therapy until she was navigating independently. The recovery had interrupted her Step Two diet, and so Beth returned to Step One, followed by Step Two until she reached her desired weight. She is now cane-free, pain-free, and her prediabetes is no longer an issue, as her A1C has consistently been 5.3 to 5.4!

She lives on Step Three, the maintenance phase of the Metabolism Miracle, with brief intervals of Steps One and Two to give her metabolism an occasional rest and rehab. "I rested and rehabbed my knee," she said. "The least I can do is take some R&R for my metabolism!"

Jen L., the Soon-to-Be College Athlete, Needs Help to Get in the Game!

When Jen first came to my practice it was April of her senior year in high school. A good student and star player for the varsity softball team, Jenny was a bubbly, friendly, outgoing young woman with a bright future.

At five-foot-six and weighing 160 pounds, Jen's physical activity included lifting weights to strengthen her arms and her core and doing aerobic activity to increase her stamina. She looked much thinner than her scale weight, was in great shape, and had never thought about dieting.

After softball season Jen was taking some time off to relax before getting ready to go to college. Over time, however, Jen began to feel run down after even a short bout of exercise. Her once-strong and toned muscles were covered with a thin layer of fat, and her bikini showed a small roll around her middle. She had trouble sleeping, had difficulty getting out of bed before 11 a.m., needed a nap in the afternoon, and left her friends early in the evening to go home and sleep.

Jen knew precollege training was a necessity. Her coach had sent a training packet, and she was already two weeks behind. She also noticed that her period had become erratic. She experienced wicked PMS, and her once clean and clear face now had acne. All in all, Jen looked and felt like a different person.

Her family doctor tested her for PCOS, hypothyroidism, and anemia, but Beth's physical exam was pretty normal. The next day she found out she did have PCOS, her cholesterol was higher than last year, and her blood pressure had risen a bit too.

Her mom decided Jen should have a registered dietitian review her diet. When she walked in the door, I couldn't quite figure what I was seeing her for. She looked like a typical college student, did not look overweight or out of shape, but did seem withdrawn and sad.

I took a look at her fasting lab work and saw a few things. Her LDL cholesterol was in the Met B range. So was her glucose and vitamin D level. Jen was what I would call pre-metabolism B. Her labs and blood pressure plus physical symptoms showed she had just stepped on the Met B train.

When I weighed and measured Jen, even I was surprised to see the scale at 162 pounds. "That's two pounds heavier than graduation day just a few weeks ago," she told me.

Seeing her weight was the clincher. Jen was "all in."

I saw her four weeks later for a short visit just to check on how she was doing. Her skin was already clearer, and I could see her muscle tone. She still mentioned feeling fatigued, especially after her workout. I explained

Fueling Forward for her one- to one-and-a-half-hour workouts, and she was thrilled to know she could get in an energy-fueling "treat."

We met again right before she left for school. She was losing weight and inches right on target. She looked alive, healthy, and was smiling—a lot.

I was happy to see Jen had contacted her new school and asked for a few menus: yep, Step One and Step Two could easily be followed in college!

18

The Power
of Positive Thinking

I feel compelled to mention the power of positive thinking in a book that is about improved health, fat loss, and well-being.

A negative mindset sets the stage for a negative outcome. If you think you will fail, you will fail. This is why you may need to make a conscious effort to reframe your thoughts and point your mindset toward success.

Most people who begin MM start the lifestyle feeling pretty crummy. They feel some combination of exhausted, frustrated, untrusting, anxious, depressed, and unmotivated. They are tired of trying to lose weight only to regain it all. They've developed an aversion to scales, tape measures, measuring cups, food scales, swimsuit season, clothes shopping, and registered dietitians.

During our initial session most new patients cry. Sometimes I cry right along with them. I can empathize with anyone suffering with uncontrolled Met B. I know they don't look the way they want, feel the way they want, are not as healthy as they want, and are tired of living with deprivation and nothing to show for all their hard work. The longer they've lived with uncontrolled Met B, the worse they feel.

When I explain Metabolism B and its impact on health, energy, body size, and energy levels, they see a ray of hope. I can tell when an invisible lightbulb switches on and they get it for the first time. There *is* a solution, and they are ready to embrace this program developed for their situation.

This program is unlike anything you've ever seen or tried. It is an *original* program designed to seamlessly match Metabolism B. For the first time in a long time you will eat in line with your metabolism instead of against it. Take a leap of faith with this program or take a look at anyone you know who is living the Metabolism Miracle. This program works. Period.

I am now a firm believer that your mind and thoughts consciously or subconsciously form and impact the outcome of every day of your life. If you tell yourself, *It'll never work. I will never lose this weight. Why bother?* you may never make it through the first five days of Step One. You will have shut the door of permanent success before you take your first step through the door.

I suggest that you consciously feed yourself a steady diet of positive outcomes. After developing this habit, your positive mindset will become the way you see the world.

Engage in self-talk like:

"This program is written for *me*, and it will work for *me*."
"I can finally control my weight."
"I am in control."
"I am getting, feeling, and looking healthy."
"I am burning away excess body fat."
"I look younger and healthier."
"I am strong."
"I can and will do this."
"I will do this for me because I deserve all it will enable."

Focusing on these positive affirmations will strengthen your conviction, and before you know it, you will honestly believe in a positive outcome.

I find it helpful to say my positive affirmations aloud, three times in succession, several times a day so I can hear what I'm saying and really register it. I say my affirmations when I wake up, when I'm driving, when I'm taking a break at work, and before bed. Take the time to focus on the words you are saying. Try to finish the affirmation with a positive nod.

Some people post their personal positive affirmations throughout their house or office with little sticky notes on their bathroom mirror, makeup area, refrigerator, or on the dash of the car. They are reminders of the great results they *will* have.

The more often you tell yourself positive thoughts, the more you will believe the words and feel the positive energy slowly but surely changing the way you see the world. Before you fall asleep at night and the very first thing in the morning, speak confidently and positively to yourself.

Say this . . .	Instead of this . . .
"I am getting thinner and healthier every day."	"I don't see anything happening."
"I am doing this very well."	"I hope I can do this."
"I feel so much more alive and energetic."	"I feel twice my age."
"I am a success."	"I have always failed."
"The Metabolism Miracle will work for me because it was designed for me."	"I hope this works."
"I can feel my energy returning."	"I'm so tired."
"My clothes are getting looser every day."	"I look heavy in this outfit."
"It will take time to get to where I want to be, and I will stay there."	"Why is this taking so long? How can I speed this up?"

When you fill your mind and life with positive thoughts they will overflow into a positive way of living. The Metabolism Miracle starts a new beginning to your life. Expect it to work for you, know it will work for you, and watch it work for you. For the first time in a long time you will work with your metabolism instead of against it, and you will be in tune with your mind, body, and soul.

PART FOUR

Recipes

Breakfast

Easy Egg Cups

For Steps One, Two, and Three; COUNT AS NEUTRAL.

SERVES 4

---

4 ounces shredded low-fat cheese

8 strips cooked turkey bacon, finely chopped

4 whole eggs

Salt and pepper

4 tablespoons light cream

4 tablespoons grated Parmesan cheese

1. Preheat the oven to 350°F. Spray the bottoms and sides of 4 cups of a muffin tin with cooking spray.
2. Drop 1 ounce of the cheese into each cup. Place one-quarter of the chopped turkey bacon in each cup. Break one egg into each cup, leaving whole.
3. Add salt and pepper to the cream, mix well, and pour 1 tablespoon into each cup. Sprinkle the top of each cup with 1 tablespoon of grated Parmesan. Bake for 10 minutes. If desired, brown the cheese under the broiler for an additional 2 to 3 minutes. Serve warm.

Healthy "McMiracle" Muffin

For Steps Two and Three; 11 TO 20-GRAM CARB DAM, OR ONE CARB SERVING.

SERVES 1

---

1 or 2 eggs
Salt and pepper to taste
¼ cup low fat grated Cheddar cheese
1 toasted multigrain light English muffin
1 slice cooked Canadian bacon

1. Spray a medium fry pan with cooking spray and place over medium heat.
2. Whisk 1 or 2 eggs with salt and pepper in a small mixing bowl. Pour the eggs into the fry pan, and cook for about 2 minutes. Top the eggs with cheese, cover, and allow cheese to melt.
3. Toast the English muffin. Place the Canadian bacon on the toasted muffin, add the eggs, and enjoy!

Sunshine Breakfast Sandwich

For Steps One, Two, and Three; 5 GRAM COUNTER CARB, OR 5 GRAMS NET CARB.

SERVES 1

---

1 slice low-carb whole-grain bread (5 or fewer grams net carb)
1 teaspoon whipped or softened butter
1 egg
Salt and pepper to taste

1. Spray a small fry pan with cooking spray and heat over medium-high heat.
2. Spread the butter over the bread. Use a small cookie cutter or the top of a glass to cut out the middle of the bread, then place the outside of the cut-out bread, butter side down, in the fry pan.
3. Crack one egg into a cup, and then gently pour into the hole in the center of the bread. Add salt and pepper to taste, and cook the egg to your

preference (usually about 3 minutes). For a well-done egg, flip the egg and bread over and cook for an additional 1 minute or less.

4. Serve the egg yolk side up so the "sunshine" greets you!

Egg Taco

For Steps One, Two, and Three; 5 GRAM COUNTER CARB, OR 5 GRAMS NET CARB.

SERVES 1

---

1 or 2 eggs (or ½ cup egg whites or egg substitute)

2 tablespoons half-and-half

Salt and pepper to taste

1 low-carb tortilla (5 or fewer grams net carb)

2 tablespoons shredded Cheddar cheese

1 teaspoon guacamole

1 tablespoon regular or light sour cream

Salsa to taste

1. Spray a small fry pan with cooking spray and heat over medium heat.
2. Whisk the eggs with half-and-half in a small mixing bowl, and season with salt and pepper. Pour into the heated fry pan and cook to desired doneness.
3. Place the cooked eggs into the tortilla, top with cheese, guacamole, sour cream, and salsa. Fold and enjoy!

Miracle Quiche

For Steps One, Two, and Three; COUNT AS NEUTRAL.

SERVES 4

---

1 tablespoon butter

½ medium onion, diced

2 cups sliced mushrooms

1 cup diced fresh broccoli florets

½ cup half-and-half or light cream

4 ounces grated low-fat Cheddar cheese

Salt and pepper to taste

6 eggs, beaten

1. Preheat the oven to 325°F. Spray the bottom and sides of a 9-inch ceramic or glass pie pan with cooking spray.
2. Melt the butter in a skillet, and sauté the onion, mushrooms, and broccoli until onions are golden and broccoli is al dente.
3. Meanwhile, heat the half-and-half in a medium saucepan over medium heat until just below boiling. Remove from the heat and stir in the cheese until it melts. Add the vegetables and salt and pepper to the cheese mixture. Mix well and let cool for 5 minutes.
4. Add the beaten eggs to the mixture, and mix well. Pour into the prepared pie pan, and bake for 45 to 50 minutes, until the custard is set or a knife inserted into the center of the quiche comes out clean. Cool on a rack for at least 5 minutes before slicing.

Crustless Ham, Cheddar, and Veggie Quiche

For Steps One, Two, and Three; COUNT AS NEUTRAL.

SERVES 4

½ pound ham, diced into small cubes

8 ounces low-fat or regular shredded Cheddar cheese

1 large fresh tomato, seeded and diced

10 ounces frozen chopped spinach, completely thawed, with excess liquid squeezed out

2 tablespoons butter

2 teaspoons olive oil

1 medium onion, finely chopped

½ green bell pepper, seeded and finely chopped

1 cup sliced mushrooms

6 eggs, beaten

½ cup light cream or half-and-half

¼ teaspoon salt

⅛ teaspoon black pepper

1. Preheat the oven to 350°F. Lightly coat a 9-inch glass or ceramic pie plate with cooking spray. Distribute the ham, cheese, tomato, and spinach in the bottom of the pie plate.
2. Heat the butter and oil in a skillet. Add the onion, bell pepper, and mushrooms, and sauté until the onions turn glossy and are tender; spread the vegetable mixture into the pie plate.
3. Using the same skillet, stir together the eggs, cream, salt, and pepper, and heat for 5 minutes, stirring constantly. Pour the cooked eggs over the ham, cheese, and vegetable base.
4. Bake for approximately 50 minutes, or until a knife inserted into the center of the quiche comes out clean. Cool on a rack for at least 5 minutes before slicing.

Sun-Dried Tomato and Spinach Omelet

For Steps One, Two, and Three; COUNT AS NEUTRAL.

SERVES 1

½ cup egg whites or egg substitute or 2 whole eggs

2 tablespoons half-and-half or light cream

Salt and pepper to taste

¼ cup low-fat cottage cheese or ricotta

½ cup chopped baby spinach

2 tablespoons chopped sun-dried tomatoes

1. Spray a medium fry pan with cooking spray, and heat on medium-high.
2. Whisk together the egg whites, half-and-half, and salt and pepper in a small mixing bowl. Pour the egg mixture into the fry pan, and turn pan so it spreads out evenly. When eggs begin to set, spread with the cottage cheese, spinach, and sun-dried tomatoes.
3. Fold the omelet in half and cook 2 more minutes, or until eggs are to your preference of doneness and the cheese is melted.

Vegan Breakfast Scramble

For Steps One, Two, and Three; COUNT AS NEUTRAL.

SERVES 1

---

1 teaspoon olive oil

½ cup diced firm tofu

¼ cup baby spinach

2 tablespoons chopped red or green bell pepper

2 tablespoons chopped onion

2 tablespoons cooked vegetarian bacon, chopped

Salt and pepper to taste

Prepare a medium fry pan with cooking spray and heat over medium-high. Add 1 teaspoon of the oil. Add the tofu, spinach, peppers, onion, bacon, and salt and pepper; sauté until the onions are golden, the vegetables are cooked, and the tofu is lightly browned, about 10–15 minutes.

Easy Pizza

For Steps One, Two, and Three;

COUNTS AS 5-GRAM COUNTER CARB OR 5 GRAMS NET CARB.

SERVES 1

---

1 slice low-carb bread (5 or fewer grams net carb), toasted

1 slice mozzarella cheese

2 tablespoons ricotta or cottage cheese

2 slices fresh tomato

½ teaspoon of olive oil

Grated Parmesan cheese

⅛ teaspoon Italian seasoning

Salt and pepper to taste

1. Preheat the broiler (or toaster oven broiler).
2. Place the toast on a baking tray lined with parchment paper. Top with the mozzarella, spread on the ricotta, add the tomato, and drizzle

with the olive oil. Sprinkle the Parmesan on top, and add the Italian seasoning and salt and pepper.

3. Broil until the cheese is melted.

Easy "Bacon" Pizza

For Steps One, Two, and Three;

5-GRAM COUNTER CARB, OR 5 GRAMS NET CARB.

SERVES 1

---

1 low-carb tortilla (5 or fewer grams net carb)

½ teaspoon olive oil

2 tablespoons low-fat ricotta cheese

2 to 3 tablespoons marinara sauce (no added sugar; check ingredients)

¼ cup shredded mozzarella cheese

¼ cup shredded provolone cheese

2 slices turkey bacon, cooked and crumbled

1 teaspoon grated Parmesan cheese

Salt and pepper to taste

1. Preheat the broiler (or toaster oven broiler).
2. Place the tortilla on a baking tray lined with parchment paper, and sprinkle with the oil. Broil for 1 minute until lightly browned.
3. Spread the ricotta over the tortilla, then follow with the marinara. Sprinkle the mozzarella and provolone on top of the marinara, then add the bacon and top with Parmesan and salt and pepper.
4. Return to broiler and cook until the cheese is melted.

Hot "Cereal"

For Steps One, Two, and Three; COUNT AS NEUTRAL.

SERVES 1

¼ cup finely chopped almonds

¼ cup finely chopped walnuts

2 tablespoons ground sesame seeds

1 teaspoon butter

¼ cup light cream or half-and-half

⅛ teaspoon ground cinnamon

One 1-gram packet Splenda

Pinch of salt to taste

1. Process the almonds, walnuts, and sesame seeds in a food processor until they are a fine consistency. Place the nut mixture in a microwave-safe cereal bowl. Add the butter, cream, cinnamon, Splenda, and salt, and mix well.
2. Microwave on HIGH for 30 seconds or until the butter is melted. Stir, close your eyes, and think "hot cereal."

Oatmeal Cup

For Steps Two and Three; 11- TO 20-GRAM CARB DAM, OR ONE CARB SERVING.

SERVES 1

¼ cup quick-cooking oats

3 tablespoons egg substitute

2 teaspoons carb-free maple syrup

2 tablespoons unsweetened vanilla almond milk

2 tablespoons almond flour

½ teaspoon vanilla extract

¼ teaspoon baking powder

⅛ teaspoon ground cinnamon

1. Spray a large microwave-safe mug with cooking spray.

2. Combine all of the ingredients in a small mixing bowl, and mix well. Pour the mixture into the prepared mug, and flatten it in.
3. Microwave on HIGH for 45 to 60 seconds. Enjoy straight out of the mug!

Silver Dollar Pancakes

For Steps One, Two, and Three; ONE SERVING COUNTS AS NEUTRAL.

MAKES 5 SERVINGS OF 6 PANCAKES

---

1 cup part-skim ricotta cheese
⅓ cup soy flour or almond flour
1 tablespoon oil
½ teaspoon vanilla extract
One 1-gram packet Splenda
Pinch of salt
4 eggs, beaten
Carb-free maple syrup, whipped butter, light whipped cream, or carb-free jelly for toppings

1. Spray a griddle pan or skillet with cooking spray, and heat on medium-high.
2. Blend together the ricotta, soy flour, oil, vanilla, Splenda, and salt in a mixing bowl. Fold in the eggs—the mixture should have a batter-like consistency.
3. Spoon the mixture onto the prepared hot skillet in silver dollar–sized spoonfuls. Lightly brown on both sides, turning only once. Continue with the rest of the batter, respraying the skillet with cooking spray between pancakes.
4. Serve with syrup, butter, light whipped cream, or a dollop of jelly.

Pumpkin Muesli

For Steps Two and Three; 11- TO 20-GRAM CARB DAM, OR ONE CARB SERVING.

SERVES 1

_____

¼ cup quick-cooking oats

¼ cup pumpkin puree (no added sugar, don't use sweetened pumpkin pie filling)

½ cup plain low-fat Greek yogurt

Stevia, sucralose, or erythritol to taste

1 teaspoon lemon zest

2 tablespoons slivered almonds

1. Lightly spray a microwave-safe bowl with cooking spray.
2. Mix together the oats and pumpkin puree in a small bowl, and pour into the microwave-safe bowl. Cover tightly with plastic wrap, and microwave on HIGH for 30 seconds.
3. Remove from microwave and let the mug sit, covered, for about 10 minutes.
4. Meanwhile, combine the yogurt, stevia, zest, and almonds. Stir the yogurt mixture into the oat mixture, and enjoy!

Fruity Yogurt Parfait

For Steps Two and Three; 11- TO 20-GRAM CARB DAM, OR ONE CARB SERVING.

SERVES 1

_____

1 cup plain Greek yogurt

1 teaspoon sucralose, stevia, or erythritol

½ teaspoon vanilla extract

4 medium strawberries, thinly sliced

½ cup blueberries

¼ cup slivered almonds

¼ cup unsweetened coconut flakes

Real whipped cream

1. Combine the yogurt, sweetener, and vanilla in a small bowl.
2. Wash and dry the berries.
3. Layer half the yogurt mixture into a clear 16-ounce glass, followed by half the almonds, half the coconut, half the strawberries, then half the blueberries. Repeat the layers, ending with the blueberries.
4. Top with a swirl of whipped cream.

Chocolate Strawberry Protein Smoothie

For Steps One, Two, and Three; 5-GRAM COUNTER CARB.

SERVES 1

---

1 cup unsweetened chocolate almond milk
¼ cup strawberry slices
½ packet Splenda or stevia
Scoop unflavored whey protein powder
4 ice cubes

Place all of the ingredients into a blender, and mix until smooth.

Fruited Yogurt Smoothie

For Steps Two and Three; 11- TO 20-GRAM CARB DAM, OR ONE CARB SERVING.

SERVES 1

---

4 small strawberries
¼ cup blueberries
¾ cup plain Greek yogurt
1 packet sucralose or stevia
¼ cup unsweetened vanilla almond milk
4 ice cubes

Place all of the ingredients into a blender, and mix until smooth.

Broiled Grapefruit and Ricotta

For Steps Two and Three; 11- TO 20-GRAM CARB DAM, OR ONE CARB SERVING.

SERVES 1

½ medium grapefruit, chilled

Erythritol, sucralose, or stevia to taste

Light sprinkle of salt

½ cup low-fat ricotta cheese

Dash of ground cinnamon

Dash of ground nutmeg

1. Preheat the broiler (or toaster oven broiler).
2. Place the grapefruit face up on a baking tray lined with parchment paper. Sprinkle with sweetener and salt to taste.
3. Broil for 3 to 4 minutes. Serve with the ricotta mixed with cinnamon and nutmeg.

Appetizers and Snacks

Clam and Crab Cold Dip

For Steps One, Two, and Three; COUNT AS NEUTRAL.

MAKES APPROXIMATELY 2½ CUPS DIP

One 8-ounce package cream cheese (regular or light)

¼ cup olive oil

¼ cup mayonnaise (light or regular)

One 6½-ounce can minced crabmeat, drained

One 6½-ounce can minced clams, drained

Salt and pepper

2 tablespoons finely chopped fresh dill or 1 teaspoon dried dill weed

¼ cup finely chopped fresh parsley or 2 teaspoons dried parsley flakes

¼ teaspoon garlic powder

¼ teaspoon onion powder

¼ teaspoon of Old Bay seasoning

1 splash hot sauce, optional

1. Combine all of the the ingredients in a medium saucepan over low heat, stirring occasionally for 30 minutes until thoroughly warmed.
2. Transfer to a container, cover with a lid or plastic wrap, and chill overnight.
3. Serve as a dip for neutral veggies such as green or red bell peppers, cauliflower, broccoli, mushrooms, or whole green beans.

Veggie Mini-Pizza

For Steps One, Two, and Three; 5-GRAM COUNTER CARB.

SERVES 4

---

4 low-carb tortillas (5 or fewer grams net carb each)
½ cup marinara sauce (no added sugar; check ingredients)
¼ cup Classic Pesto (page 279, or use jarred)
¼ cup finely chopped broccoli florets
1 cup baby spinach
16 mushrooms, cleaned and sliced
¼ cup finely chopped sweet onion
Sliced olives, optional
1 cup shredded mozzarella

1. Preheat the broiler (or toaster oven broiler). Line a baking tray with parchment paper.
2. Place the tortillas on the baking tray. Spread the marinara over each tortilla, then top with pesto. Sprinkle the remaining ingredients evenly over each tortilla.
3. Broil until cheese is melted.

Feta-Stuffed Mushrooms

For Steps One, Two, and Three; COUNT AS NEUTRAL.

SERVES 2

---

2 portobello mushrooms (5 to 6 ounces each)
Oil from sun-dried tomatoes (below)
One 4-ounce package crumbled feta cheese
½ cup chopped pitted ripe olives
2 tablespoons chopped, oil-packed sun-dried tomatoes

1. Preheat the oven to 425°F. Coat a baking sheet with cooking spray.
2. Remove and discard the mushroom stems. Clean the mushrooms, and place the mushroom caps, underside up, on the baking sheet; brush

the inside of each mushroom with the sundried tomato oil, and set aside.

3. Combine the cheese, olives, and sundried tomatoes in a small mixing bowl, and mix well. Divide the cheese mixture equally, and place atop each of the mushrooms.

4. Bake for 10 minutes, or until completely heated. Serve warm.

Buffalo "Wings," Cauliflower Style

For Steps One, Two, and Three; COUNT AS NEUTRAL.

SERVES 4 TO 6

---

1 cup unsweetened almond milk

1 cup almond flour

2 teaspoons garlic powder

1 teaspoon onion powder

¼ teaspoon black pepper

1 head fresh cauliflower, chopped

1 cup buffalo sauce (bottled is fine)

Light blue cheese dressing

1. Preheat the oven to 400°F. Line a baking sheet with parchment paper and set aside.

2. Whisk together the almond milk, almond flour, garlic powder, onion powder, and pepper in a large mixing bowl. Let the whisked mixture sit for 10 minutes to allow the flavors to blend.

3. Add the cauliflower bites to the almond milk mixture, and mix well. Let the cauliflower rest in the mixture for 10 minutes to absorb the moisture.

4. Pick up the cauliflower pieces one at a time, shake off the excess batter, and place on the baking sheet. Bake for 15 to 20 minutes.

5. Remove from the oven, and toss in the buffalo sauce until well coated.

6. Replace parchment paper on the baking sheet, place the cauliflower back on the sheet, and bake for another 8 to 10 minutes.

7. Allow to cool slightly, and serve with blue cheese dressing for dipping.

Crispy Tortilla Chips

For Steps One, Two, and Three; 5-GRAM COUNTER CARB.

SERVES 1

---

1 low-carb tortilla (5 or fewer grams net carb)
Garlic powder to taste
Salt and pepper to taste
Grated Parmesan cheese

1. Preheat the oven to 425°F. Coat a baking sheet with cooking spray.
2. Cut the tortilla into 8 chip-size triangles, and place them on the cookie sheet. Lightly spray the tortilla triangles with cooking spray, then immediately sprinkle each with the desired amount of garlic powder, salt, pepper, and cheese.
3. Bake for 5 to 8 minutes, until golden brown and crispy. Watch periodically to make sure they don't burn. Let cool before eating.

Sweet-and-Sour Cucumbers

For Steps One, Two, and Three; COUNT AS NEUTRAL.

SERVES 6

---

2 cups unpeeled, sliced, well-washed cucumbers
1 cup very thinly sliced red onion
¼ cup white vinegar
¼ teaspoon dried dill
1 tablespoon powdered Splenda
Salt and pepper to taste

1. Mix the cucumber and onion in a medium mixing bowl.
2. Whisk together the remaining ingredients in a separate bowl.
3. Pour the sauce over the cucumbers, and chill for at least 2 hours.
4. Toss before serving. Serve chilled.

Cheesy Chips

For Steps One, Two, and Three; COUNT AS NEUTRAL.

SERVES 1

½ cup grated or shredded cheese yields 8 cheesy chips
Coarsely grated Parmesan or Cheddar cheese

1. Preheat the oven to 400°F. Coat a baking sheet with cooking spray.
2. Spoon 1 tablespoon of the cheese onto the cookie sheet, and pat down to form a little disk. Repeat for the remaining cheese.
3. Bake for 5 minutes. Let cool before removing the chips from the cookie sheet.

Sweet Walnut or Mixed Nut Treat

For Steps One, Two, and Three; COUNT AS NEUTRAL.

MAKES 2 CUPS OF NUTS (4 TO 6 SERVINGS)

---

2 tablespoons butter
2 cups walnut halves or a mixture of any nuts
½ cup granulated Splenda
1 tablespoon vanilla extract
1 tablespoon ground cinnamon
¼ teaspoon ground nutmeg

1. Melt the butter in a large skillet over medium heat. Add the nuts, and stir to coat. Add the remaining ingredients, and stir well to coat.
2. Remove nuts from the skillet, lay flat on a dish, and allow to cool. Store in an airtight container.

Ham and Cream Cheese "Packets"

For Steps One, Two, and Three; COUNT AS NEUTRAL.

SERVES 4

---

4 ounces light cream cheese, softened
¼ cup finely chopped scallions
½ teaspoon prepared horseradish, or a splash of hot sauce, optional
Salt and pepper, optional
1 pound (16 slices) thinly sliced deli ham
16 tiny pitted olives

1. Mix the cream cheese, scallions, horseradish, and salt and pepper in a small mixing bowl.
2. Lay flat a piece of ham, and place a spoonful of the cream cheese mixture in the center. Fold all sides of the ham toward the middle to form a square, top with an olive, and then secure with a toothpick. Repeat for the remaining ham and cream cheese mixture.

Sun-Dried Tomato Dip

For Steps One, Two, and Three; COUNT AS NEUTRAL.

MAKES ABOUT 2½ CUPS DIP (ABOUT 10 SERVINGS)

---

8 ounces low-fat cottage cheese
8 ounces ricotta cheese
1 finely chopped green onion
½ cup finely chopped red or green bell pepper
¼ cup finely chopped oil-packed sun-dried tomatoes
1 tablespoon fresh basil, or 1 teaspoon dried basil
1 teaspoon lemon juice
⅛ teaspoon salt
⅛ teaspoon black pepper

Combine all of the ingredients in blender or food processor; blend until smooth. Refrigerate for at least 2 hours. Serve as a dip for neutral veggies such as bell peppers, broccoli, celery, or mushrooms.

Classic Pesto

For Steps One, Two, and Three; COUNT AS NEUTRAL.

MAKES ABOUT 1½ TO 2 CUPS

⅓ cup pine nuts

3 garlic cloves, unpeeled

3 cups packed fresh basil

⅓ cup olive oil

⅓ cup grated Parmesan cheese

Salt to taste

1. Heat a skillet over medium-high heat. Add the pine nuts and garlic cloves, and toast until golden brown, shaking the pan occasionally to toss and promote an even golden color. When the nuts are golden, take them out of the skillet to cool in a single layer on a plate. Continue to toast the garlic until it is also golden, then place on the plate with the pine nuts to cool. Once cool, remove the skins from the garlic.
2. Combine the pine nuts, garlic, basil, and olive oil in a food processor; pulse until grainy in texture.
3. Transfer to a mixing bowl, and stir in the cheese and salt to taste.
4. Store in a covered jar, adding olive oil to the top of the mixture before capping. After each use add a little more olive oil to the top of the pesto to help it keep for several weeks in your refrigerator.

Sandwiches

Roast Beef with Horseradish Wrap

For Steps One, Two, and Three; 5-GRAM COUNTER CARB.

SERVES 4

---

4 ounces cream cheese

1 tablespoon horseradish

4 low-carb wraps (5 or fewer grams net carb each)

8 ounces thinly sliced or shaved roast beef

4 ounces shredded Cheddar cheese

1 cup chopped Romaine leaves

Combine the cream cheese and horseradish in a medium mixing bowl, then spread ¼ of the cream cheese mixture on top of each wrap. Next add ¼ of the roast beef, followed by the cheese and lettuce. Roll up and enjoy.

Greek-Inspired Wraps

For Steps One, Two, and Three; 5-GRAM COUNTER CARB.

SERVES 4

---

4 low-carb tortillas (5 or fewer grams net carb each)

1 cup plain Greek yogurt

1 cup chopped greens

2 large roasted red peppers, sliced

¼ cup crumbled feta

¼ cup chopped black olives

1½ cucumbers, peeled and thinly sliced

Spread each tortilla with ¼ of the yogurt. Then on each sprinkle ¼ of the greens, red pepper, feta, olives, and cucumber. Roll up and enjoy.

Ham and Pineapple Chopped Salad with Side Wrap

For Steps Two and Three; 11- TO 20-GRAM CARB DAM OR ONE CARB SERVING.

SERVES 4

---

2 cups Greek yogurt

2 tablespoons apple cider vinegar

1 tablespoon flax seeds

1 cup diced pineapple (drained if using canned)

1 cup chopped red apple

1 carrot, shredded

8 ounces deli ham, chopped

½ head sweet cabbage, shredded

4 low-carb wraps (11 to 20 grams net carb each)

1. Combine the yogurt, vinegar, and flax seeds in a small mixing bowl.
2. Mix together in a medium mixing bowl the pineapple, apple, carrot, ham, and cabbage. Then add the yogurt mixture to the pineapple mixture, and mix well. Chill salad.
3. Serve ¼ of the salad with 1 tortilla.

Miracle Grilled Cheese

For Steps One, Two, and Three; COUNT AS A 5-GRAM COUNTER CARB.

SERVES 1

---

1 teaspoon butter

1 low-carb tortilla or wrap (5 or fewer grams net carb)

½ cup shredded cheese of your choice

Coat a small nonstick skillet with cooking spray, and heat on high heat. Melt the butter in the pan, then place the tortilla on top of the melted butter, and spread the cheese across the tortilla. When the tortilla bottom is golden brown and the cheese begins to melt, flip the tortilla in half to close it up. Heat for 15 seconds on both sides. Serve warm.

Nicoise "Sandwiches"

For Steps Two and Three; 11- TO 20-GRAM CARB DAM, OR ONE CARB SERVING.

SERVES 2

_____

One 6-ounce can water-packed white tuna, drained
12 cherry tomatoes, halved
½ cup chopped black olives
4 teaspoons olive oil
Salt and pepper to taste
4 slices light whole-grain bread
1 cup baby spinach leaves

Combine the tuna, tomatoes, olives, oil, and salt and pepper in a medium mixing bowl. Spoon ½ of the tuna mixture on 2 slices of bread, spread the spinach leaves over the mixture, then top with the other slice of bread. Cut in half and enjoy.

Open-Faced Hummus and Avocado

For Steps Two and Three; 11- TO 20-GRAM CARB DAM, OR ONE CARB SERVING.

SERVES 1

_____

½ cup canned chickpeas, drained
¼ fresh avocado, pitted
1 tablespoon finely chopped parsley
1 tablespoon chopped olives
1 teaspoon olive oil
¼ teaspoon lemon juice
Salt and pepper to taste
1 slice low-carb bread (5 or fewer grams net carb), toasted

½ cup finely chopped dark greens

1 to 2 slices tomato

1 very thin slice Vidalia onion

1. Mash together in a mixing bowl the chickpeas, avocado, parsley, olives, oil, lemon juice, and salt and pepper.
2. Toast the bread, then spread the chickpea mixture over it. Top with the greens, tomato, and onion. Enjoy!

Peaches and Creamy Grilled Cheese

For Steps Two and Three; 11- TO 20-GRAM CARB DAM, OR ONE CARB SERVING.

SERVES 1

½ cup ricotta or cottage cheese

1 tablespoon whipped cream cheese

1 to 2 tablespoons carb-free peach jelly (e.g., Walden Farms™ zero-carb jelly)

¼ teaspoon lemon juice

2 slices light whole-grain bread (11- to 20-grams net carb total)

1. Combine the ricotta, cream cheese, jelly, and lemon juice in a small mixing bowl.
2. Spread the ricotta mixture across one piece of bread, then top with the other piece.
3. Coat a medium fry pan with cooking spray and heat over medium-high heat. Place the sandwich in the pan, and grill for 2 to 3 minutes per side, like a grilled cheese sandwich.

Roast Beef and Apple Quesadilla

For Steps Two and Three; 11- TO 20-GRAM CARB DAM, OR ONE CARB SERVING.

SERVES 1

---

2 tablespoons light cream cheese

1 low-carb tortilla (5 or fewer grams net carb)

3 slices thinly sliced roast beef

½ apple, thinly sliced

¼ cup shredded Cheddar cheese

1. Coat a frying pan with cooking spray and heat over medium-high heat.
2. Spread the cream cheese over the tortilla, then add the roast beef, apple, and cheese. Fold in half, and grill in the frying pan for 2 to 3 minutes on each side, turning once.

Soups and Salads

Roasted Broccoli and Cheddar Soup

Steps One, Two, or Three; COUNT AS NEUTRAL.

SERVES 4

---

1 large bunch broccoli, cut into florets
Olive oil cooking spray
Salt and pepper
1 tablespoon olive oil
1 medium onion, finely chopped
2 cloves garlic, finely chopped
3 cups vegetable or chicken broth
1 teaspoon dried dill weed
1 cup half-and-half
1½ cups aged cheddar, shredded

1. Preheat the oven 400°F.
2. Arrange the broccoli in a single layer on a large baking sheet. Lightly coat the broccoli florets with the olive oil cooking spray, and sprinkle with salt and pepper. Roast until lightly golden brown, turning occasionally, about 10 to 15 minutes.
3. Heat the oil in a large sauce pan over medium heat. Add the onion and garlic, and sauté, stirring frequently, until golden brown, about 5 to 7 minutes. Add the broth, dill, and broccoli, bring to a boil, reduce the heat, cover, and simmer for 15 minutes.
4. Gently whisk in the half-and-half and cheese until the cheese melts.
5. Puree the soup with a blender, food processor, or immersion blender.

If you make this in a slow cooker, roast the broccoli florets, then place all ingredients except the half-and-half and cheese in your slow cooker. Heat on LOW for 6 hours or on HIGH for 2 hours before mixing in the half-and-half and cheese. Once the cheese is melted, puree it into a soup.

Miracle Coleslaw

Steps One, Two, or Three; COUNT AS NEUTRAL.

SERVES 6 TO 8

One 16-ounce package coleslaw mix
¼ cup thinly sliced onions
⅓ cup Splenda sugar substitute
½ teaspoon salt
⅛ teaspoon fresh ground black pepper
½ teaspoon celery seed
½ cup light mayonnaise
¼ cup half-and-half or light cream
1½ tablespoons white vinegar
2½ tablespoons lemon juice

1. Combine the coleslaw with the onion in a large mixing bowl and set aside.
2. Whisk together in a separate bowl the remaining ingredients until very well combined. Pour over the coleslaw mix; stir gently to mix well.
3. Refrigerate for at least 2 hours before serving.

Miracle "Potato-less" Soup

For Steps One, Two, and Three; COUNT AS NEUTRAL.

SERVES 6

1 head cauliflower, broken into tiny florets
2 finely chopped scallions
1 teaspoon finely chopped garlic
4 cups chicken or vegetable broth (can be low-sodium if desired)
4 ounces light sour cream

4 ounces shredded Cheddar cheese
¼ cup butter
6 strips turkey bacon, microwaved until crisp and finely chopped
Salt and pepper to taste

1. Gently boil the cauliflower, scallions, and garlic in the broth. Check after 10 to 15 minutes to make sure the cauliflower is completely tender. Remove the cauliflower, reserving the broth, and place in a mixing bowl or food processor. Add the sour cream, cheese, and butter to the cauliflower, and mix with an immersion blender or food processor until smooth.
2. Return the cauliflower mixture to the broth. Add the bacon, and stir over medium heat. Add more broth if you prefer a thinner soup. Salt and pepper to taste.

Veggie Couscous Soup

For Steps Two and Three; 11- TO 20-GRAM CARB DAM, OR ONE CARB SERVING.

SERVES 4

---

4 cups chicken or vegetable broth
1 tablespoon olive oil
1 cup broccoli florets
2 cups cauliflower florets
1 scallion, chopped
1 cup shredded carrots
2 cups cooked couscous

1. Heat the broth and oil in a medium saucepan over medium-high heat, and bring to a boil. Add the broccoli, cauliflower, scallion, and carrots, and cook until the vegetables are tender, about 15 to 20 minutes.
2. Add the couscous to the veggies, mix, and let sit for 3 minutes before serving.

Corn Bisque

For Steps Two and Three; 11- TO 20-GRAM CARB DAM, OR ONE CARB SERVING.

SERVES 4

---

2 teaspoons olive oil

2 tablespoons finely chopped scallions

½ cup diced onion

¼ cup diced celery

2 tablespoons whole-wheat flour

2 cups frozen corn kernels

1½ cups chicken broth

½ teaspoon Worcestershire sauce

1 drop hot sauce, optional

½ teaspoon dried dill

½ teaspoon pepper

½ cup light cream or half-and-half, at room temperature

1. Heat the oil in a medium saucepan on medium-high heat. Add the scallions, onion, and celery, and stir constantly until the onion is soft and translucent.
2. Sprinkle the flour over the cooked veggies, and stir for about 2 minutes.
3. Add the remaining ingredients, except the cream, and heat for 10 minutes. Allow to cool slightly.
4. Separate ⅔ of the vegetable mixture and puree it with a blender or food processor. Return this puree back into the remaining mixture, and stir in the cream. Serve warm.

Hearty Sausage and Bean Soup

For Step One, replace the kidney beans and black beans with
2 cans white or black soy beans; COUNT AS NEUTRAL.

For Steps Two and Three; 11- TO 20-GRAM CARB DAM, OR ONE CARB SERVING.

SERVES 6 TO 8

---

1 pound ground mild Italian sausage, ground turkey sausage, or lean
    ground beef
1 cup diced onion
1 cup sliced celery
1 cup sliced carrots
One 15-ounce can red kidney beans, drained
One 15-ounce can black beans, drained
2 cups beef broth
¼ cup finely chopped fresh parsley
Two 16-ounce cans diced tomatoes
½ teaspoon salt
¼ teaspoon oregano
¼ teaspoon basil
¼ teaspoon black pepper
2 cups shredded cabbage
Parmesan cheese, optional

1. Coat a large skillet with cooking oil spray, then brown the meat; when
   cooked, drain the grease thoroughly.
2. Add the remaining ingredients, except the cabbage and cheese, and
   bring to a boil. Lower the heat, partially cover, and simmer for 30 minutes. Add the cabbage, and simmer for another 15 minutes. Garnish
   individual servings with Parmesan, if desired.

Light Chef's Salad

For Steps One, Two, and Three; COUNT AS NEUTRAL.

SERVES 4

---

1 head Romaine lettuce, rinsed, dried, and torn into bite-size pieces

2 tomatoes, sliced

2 avocados, peeled and diced

4 ounces medium-sliced deli turkey, rolled and cut into slices making pinwheels

4 ounces medium-sliced deli baked ham, rolled and cut into slices making pinwheels

4 ounces medium-sliced provolone cheese, rolled and cut into slices making pinwheels

½ thinly sliced red onion

4 hard-boiled eggs, cut in half lengthwise

⅓ cup olive oil

⅓ cup balsamic vinegar

Salt and pepper to taste

Arrange Romaine on each of four salad plates. Top each with tomato, avocado, turkey, ham, provolone, and onion. Place two egg halves on each plate. Finish with oil, vinaigrette, and salt and pepper to taste.

Tender Spinach Salad

For Steps One, Two, and Three; COUNT AS NEUTRAL.

SERVES 4

---

10 ounces fresh baby spinach, washed and dried

1 cup fresh mushroom slices

4 hard-boiled eggs, chopped

12 slices turkey bacon, cooked and chopped

½ cup olive oil

½ cup lite sour cream

¼ cup red wine vinegar

½ teaspoon dry mustard

Salt and pepper to taste

1. Toss the spinach, mushrooms, eggs, and bacon in a large bowl.
2. Whisk together in a separate mixing bowl the remaining ingredients, add the dressing to the veggies, and toss to coat.

Potato-ish Salad

For Steps One, Two, and Three; COUNT AS NEUTRAL.

SERVES 4 TO 6

1 head cauliflower, broken into small florets

½ cup light mayonnaise

½ cup light cream or half-and-half

¼ teaspoon mustard (spicy preferred)

¼ teaspoon celery seeds

1 teaspoon powdered Splenda

½ onion, very finely chopped

½ green bell pepper, very finely chopped

2 hard-boiled eggs, diced, optional

Salt and pepper to taste

1. Cook the cauliflower in a large pot of boiling salted water. Check for tenderness after 12 minutes; the cauliflower pieces should be soft, the texture of cooked potatoes for potato salad. Drain in a colander and gently pat dry.
2. Whisk together in a large mixing bowl the mayonnaise, cream, mustard, celery seeds, and Splenda. Add the cauliflower, onion, peppers, and eggs to the dressing, and toss lightly to coat. Add salt and pepper to taste. Refrigerate for at least 2 hours before serving.

Cold Pea Salad

For Steps Two and Three; 11- TO 20-GRAM CARB DAM, OR ONE CARB SERVING.

SERVES 4

---

2 cups frozen peas, thawed and dried
½ cup light sour cream
½ cup plain yogurt
¾ cup chopped scallions
Salt and pepper to taste

1. Place the peas in a bowl. Set aside.
2. Whisk together in a separate medium mixing bowl the remaining ingredients. Pour the dressing over the peas, and mix well. Cover and refrigerate at least two hours, and serve chilled.

Chunky Chicken Salad

For Steps One, Two, and Three; COUNT AS NEUTRAL.

SERVES 4

½ cup light sour cream
½ cup light mayonnaise
2 tablespoons fresh lemon juice
½ teaspoon salt
¼ teaspoon black pepper
2 cups cooked and cubed boneless, skinless chicken breast
½ green bell pepper, chopped
½ red onion, chopped
¼ cup finely chopped fresh dill
¼ cup finely chopped fresh parsley
½ cup pitted, sliced black olives, optional

1. Combine in a medium mixing bowl the sour cream, mayonnaise, lemon juice, salt, and pepper. Blend well.
2. Add the chicken, green pepper, onion, dill, parsley, and olives, and mix well. Refrigerate for at least 2 hours before serving.

Pasta Primavera Salad

For Steps Two and Three; 11- TO 20-GRAM CARB DAM, OR ONE CARB SERVING.

SERVES 10

---

1 cup diced carrots

1 cup diced yellow squash

1 cup diced red onion

1 cup small cauliflower florets

1 cup small broccoli florets

1 cup light ranch dressing

2 cups cooked whole-wheat pasta shapes

½ cup grated Parmesan cheese

1 cup diced fresh tomato

1. Steam all of the vegetables, except the tomato, until crisp-tender.
2. Transfer to a large mixing bowl, mix with the ranch dressing, and marinate for several hours in the refrigerator.
3. Mix the marinated veggies with the cooked pasta until well coated. Add the cheese and tomato, and mix thoroughly. Refrigerate for about 2 hours, and serve chilled.

Chilled Avocado Pasta Salad

For Steps One, Two, and Three; COUNT AS NEUTRAL.

SERVES 4

Two 3.5-ounce packages Konjac, Miracle, or shirataki macaroni

2 teaspoons lemon juice

1 teaspoon minced garlic

2 tablespoons olive oil

2 avocados

2 tablespoons Classic Pesto (page 279)

Salt and pepper to taste

1. Rinse the macaroni in cold water in a colander for about 2 minutes, pat dry with paper towels, and set aside.

2. Add the remaining ingredients in a food processor, and puree until smooth.
3. Toss the pasta and sauce together in a bowl, and season with salt and pepper to taste. Refrigerate for at least 2 hours, and serve chilled.

Three-Bean Salad

For Steps Two and Three; 11- TO 20-GRAM CARB DAM, OR ONE CARB SERVING.
SERVES 10

One 14-ounce can cut green beans, drained
One 14-ounce can kidney beans, drained
One 14-ounce can chickpeas (garbanzo beans), drained
1 medium red onion, finely chopped
½ cup white vinegar
¼ cup olive oil
3 tablespoons powdered Splenda
¼ teaspoon salt
¼ teaspoon pepper

1. Combine in a large mixing bowl the beans with the onion, and mix well.
2. Whisk together in a separate small mixing bowl the vinegar, oil, Splenda, salt, and pepper. Pour the dressing over the beans, and mix. Refrigerate for at least 2 hours before serving.

Spicy Salad

For Steps One, Two, and Three; COUNT AS NEUTRAL.
SERVES 4

½ cup salsa
¼ cup Greek yogurt
1 tablespoon olive oil
1 teaspoon chili powder, or more if desired
3 cups baby spinach, chopped

¼ Vidalia onion, finely chopped

¼ cup sliced black olives

4 hard-boiled eggs, chopped

1. Combine in a small mixing bowl the salsa, yogurt, oil, and chili powder. Refrigerate for at least 30 minutes.
2. Place the remaining ingredients in a bowl, and toss with the chilled dressing before serving.

Miracle "Faux-Tato" Salad

For Steps One, Two, and Three; COUNT AS NEUTRAL.

SERVES 6

---

1 head cauliflower, chopped

⅓ cup low-fat mayonnaise

⅓ cup low-fat sour cream

½ cup low-fat shredded Cheddar

6 slices turkey bacon, browned and crumbled

1 bunch green onions, chopped

Salt and pepper to taste

1. Place the cauliflower in a microwave-safe bowl with ½ cup of water; cover and microwave on HIGH for 10 minutes. Drain in a colander and set aside. (The colander should still be warm when mixed!)
2. Mix together in a large mixing bowl the mayonnaise, sour cream, cheese, bacon, and onions. Add the warm cauliflower to the dressing, and toss to coat. Taste for seasoning, and add salt and pepper to taste, tossing lightly after each addition. Cover and refrigerate for at least 2 hours before serving.

Chicken Salad with Curry

For Steps One, Two, and Three; 5-GRAM COUNTER CARB.

SERVES 4

¾ cup plain Greek yogurt

½ teaspoon curry powder, or more if desired

2 cups diced grilled chicken breast

⅓ cup finely chopped Vidalia onion

8 grapes, halved

½ apple, chopped

¼ cup chopped cilantro

2 cups chopped greens

Combine the yogurt with the curry powder in a medium mixing bowl; mix well. Add the chicken, onion, grapes, apple, and cilantro. Serve atop a handful of greens.

Quinoa Salad

For Steps Two and Three; 11- TO 20-GRAM CARB DAM, OR ONE CARB SERVING.

SERVES 4

---

2 cups cooked quinoa*, fluffed

¼ cup chopped bell pepper

¼ cup finely chopped sweet onion

1 cup rinsed and drained soy beans

¼ cup chopped parsley

¼ cup olive oil

1½ tablespoons lemon juice

Salt and pepper to taste

Mix together all of the ingredients in a medium mixing bowl, and salt and pepper to taste.

Remember to rinse the quinoa before boiling.

Entrées

Lemony Dill Chicken

For Steps One, Two, and Three; COUNT AS NEUTRAL.

SERVES 4

Salt and pepper
4 boneless, skinless chicken breasts (1 to 1¼ pounds)
2 tablespoons olive oil
½ cup finely chopped onion
2 garlic cloves, minced
1 cup reduced-sodium chicken broth
2 teaspoons flour
2 tablespoons chopped dill
1 tablespoon lemon juice

1. Salt and pepper both sides of the chicken. Heat 1 tablespoon of the oil in a large heavy skillet over medium-high heat, add the chicken, and sear until well browned on both sides, about 3 minutes per side. Transfer the chicken to a plate.
2. Reduce the heat to medium, and add the remaining 1 tablespoon of oil. Add the onion and garlic, and cook, while stirring, for 2 to 3 minutes, until onions look opaque.
3. Whisk together in a medium mixing bowl the broth, flour, 1 tablespoon of dill, and the lemon juice, and add to the pan. Cook, while whisking, until slightly thickened, about 3 minutes.
4. Return the chicken to the pan plus any accumulated juices; reduce the heat to low, and simmer until the chicken is cooked through, about 4 to 5 minutes.

5. Transfer the chicken to a warmed platter. Season the sauce with salt and pepper to taste, and spoon it over the chicken. Garnish with the remaining 1 tablespoon of dill.

Miracle Zero-Carb Pasta, Turkey, and Veggie Bake

For Steps One, Two, or Three; COUNT AS NEUTRAL.

SERVES 4

Two 7- or 8-ounce bags shirataki or Miracle Noodles
2 tablespoons olive oil
1 pound lean (97%) ground turkey
½ teaspoon salt
¼ teaspoon pepper, plus more to taste
2 tablespoons minced garlic
½ cup white wine
1 jar marinara sauce (no sugar added, just tomatoes, herbs, spices)
1 cup cubed zucchini
1 cup sliced mushrooms
1 to 1½ cups shredded light mozzarella cheese
¼ cup grated Parmesan cheese

1. Preheat the oven to 350°F. Coat a baking casserole dish with cooking spray.
2. Open and place the two packages of noodles in a colander, and rinse very well for over 2 minutes with cold water. Pat dry with paper towels, place in a large skillet, and dry cook for about 2 minutes until they are warm, turning all the while, to remove any excess water from the rinsing process. Remove from the pan, and place in a mixing bowl.
3. Add 1 tablespoon of the oil to the same large skillet, and heat over medium heat. Add the turkey, salt, pepper, and garlic. Break the turkey apart while it is cooking. When the turkey is no longer pink and is fully cooked, drain well in a colander, pressing the turkey against the sides to remove all of the grease.

4. Put the turkey back in the skillet, and add the wine and marinara sauce; heat through. Next add the zucchini, mushrooms, and the remaining 1 tablespoon of oil; cook over medium heat for 10 minutes. Add the noodles to the pot, and mix well.

5. Transfer the turkey mixture from the skillet into the casserole, top with about 1 cup of the mozzarella and ¼ cup of the Parmesan. Bake for about 15 minutes or until the cheese is melted—zero-carb "pasta"!

Shirataki, or Miracle Noodles, are made of Konjac and can be found in the refrigerator section by the tofu. They are a very low-carb product! These noodles are already "cooked" and are packed in water. Be sure not to smell them until they are rinsed and patted dry!

Whole-Wheat Pasta with Chicken Sausage Ragu

For Steps Two and Three;

HIGH-IMPACT 11- TO 20-GRAM CARB DAM, OR ONE CARB SERVING.

SERVES 4

---

3 tablespoons olive oil
½ cup chopped onion
½ cup chopped green bell pepper
1 tablespoon minced garlic
8 uncooked chicken sausage links, casings removed
3 cups canned crushed tomatoes
1 teaspoon Italian seasoning
Salt
¼ teaspoon black pepper
2 cups cooked whole-grain rigatoni

1. Heat the oil in a large fry pan over medium-high heat, and add the onion, bell peppers, and garlic; sauté until golden. Add the sausage, and continue sautéing until it is fully cooked, about 15 minutes, continually breaking the sausage meat apart with a fork as it cooks.

2. Add the tomatoes, Italian seasoning, and salt and pepper, and bring

close to boiling. Reduce the heat, and cook for about 30 minutes, partially covered.

3. Ladle the sauce over the rigatoni and serve!

You can use konjac or shirataki pasta in place of the whole-grain rigatoni, and this switch will render the entrée neutral!

Flavorful Turkey Burgers

For Steps One, Two, and Three; COUNT AS NEUTRAL.
SERVES 4 TO 5

¾ pound lean ground turkey
¼ pound ground turkey sausage
1 garlic clove, finely chopped
½ cup finely chopped onion
¼ cup grated bell pepper
2 eggs, beaten
Salt and pepper to taste
1 cup shredded Cheddar cheese

1. Combine all of the ingredients in a large mixing bowl. Wearing plastic gloves, hand mix the ingredients well.
2. Form burgers to the size you prefer, and grill them on your outdoor or indoor countertop grill, or broil until they are cooked to your individual preference.

Springtime Stir Fry . . .
Choose Chicken, Shrimp, or Tofu!

For Steps One, Two, and Three; COUNT AS NEUTRAL.
SERVES 4

---

2 tablespoons olive oil
16 asparagus spears, cut in 3 pieces each
½ cup chopped onion

2 cups snap peas

1 cup shredded carrots

2 cups tiny broccoli florets

¼ cup rice vinegar

2 packets Splenda

1 teaspoon ground ginger

2 scallions, finely chopped

2 cups cooked diced chicken breast, or 24 deveined cooked shrimp, or 2
cups firm browned tofu

1. Heat the oil in a medium skillet or wok over medium heat. Add the
   asparagus, onion, peas, carrots, and broccoli, and stir-fry for about 10
   minutes.
2. Mix together in a separate bowl the vinegar, Splenda, ginger, and scallions. Add to the cooked vegetables, and cook 5 minutes longer.
3. Stir in your choice of protein, mix well, and serve.

Spicy Shrimp and Zucchini

For Steps Two and Three; COUNT AS NEUTRAL.

SERVES 4

3 tablespoons olive oil

1 teaspoon crushed red pepper flakes (dry spice)

1 onion, finely chopped

1 red bell pepper, chopped, patted dry

2 cups thinly sliced zucchini

1½ pounds shelled and deveined uncooked shrimp

1. Heat the oil in a large skillet over medium-high heat. Add the red pepper flakes, onion, and bell pepper, and sauté for 8 minutes.
2. Add the zucchini, and cook for 8 minutes.
3. Add the shrimp, and cook for an additional 8 minutes, or until shrimp
   are opaque. Serve in individual bowls.

Tropical Salsa Scallops

For Steps Two and Three; 11- TO 20-GRAM CARB DAM, OR ONE CARB SERVING.

SERVES 4

---

4 ripe peaches, peeled and chopped
2 small cucumbers, peeled and chopped
1 tablespoon lemon juice
1 tablespoon lime juice
¼ cup Greek yogurt
¼ cup finely chopped cilantro
1½ pounds sea scallops
Salt and pepper to taste
¼ cup olive oil
3 cups Cauliflower Rice (page 321)
Unsweetened coconut flakes as garnish

1. Mix together thoroughly the peaches, cucumbers, citrus juices, yogurt, and cilantro in a large mixing bowl. Cover and refrigerate.
2. Season the scallops with salt and pepper.
3. Heat the oil in a skillet over medium-high heat, add the scallops, and sear for about 4 minutes per side, or until lightly browned and cooked through.
4. Serve the scallops with the Cauliflower Rice on the side and the peach salsa, and sprinkle with coconut flakes.

Chicken Paprikash

For Steps One, Two, and Three; COUNT AS NEUTRAL.

SERVES 4 TO 6

¼ cup olive oil
2 garlic cloves, sliced
3 pounds skinless chicken parts (legs, thighs, or breast)
Salt and pepper to taste
1 small green bell pepper, chopped

2 tablespoons paprika

1 cup chicken broth, plus extra as needed for desired consistency

½ teaspoon onion powder

8 ounces sliced mushrooms

1 cup light sour cream

1. Heat the oil and garlic in a large saucepan over medium heat until the garlic browns; remove and discard the garlic.
2. Sprinkle the chicken with salt and pepper on both sides. Add the chicken, bell peppers, paprika, broth, and onion powder, reduce the heat to low, and cook for 30 minutes.
3. Add the mushrooms, and continue to cook until the chicken is tender, about 15 more minutes, adding more broth as needed to maintain the level of liquid during cooking.
4. Remove the chicken from the mixture, and transfer to a platter.
5. Stir the sour cream into the mixture, and add enough broth to make a gravy-like consistency. Pour the gravy over the chicken, and serve hot.

Spaghetti Squash "Spaghetti"

For Steps One, Two, and Three; COUNT AS NEUTRAL.

SERVES 4 TO 6

1 spaghetti squash, cut in half, seeds removed and discarded

1 pound lean ground turkey or lean ground beef

2 garlic cloves, minced

½ cup chopped onion

½ cup chopped green bell pepper

2 jars marinara sauce (no sugar added, just tomatoes, herbs, spices)

½ cup white wine

1 cup grated Parmesan cheese

1. Place the zucchini, face down, in a microwave-safe dish with a ½-inch depth of water on the bottom. Cover with plastic wrap, make a few slits for ventilation, and microwave on HIGH until tender, about 30 minutes.

2. Coat a large skillet with cooking spray, and then cook, over medium heat, the turkey, garlic, onion, and bell pepper for about 15 to 20 minutes, breaking the turkey apart as it cooks, until the turkey is browned.
3. Add the marinara and wine, and simmer for about 30 minutes more.
4. After the squash is cooked and has cooled enough to handle, pull/shred it with a fork into a large bowl. It will actually look like strands of spaghetti!
5. Divide the "spaghetti" among four to six plates, top with the sauce, and sprinkle with Parmesan.

Chicken Scampi Miracle Pasta

For Steps One, Two, and Three; COUNT AS NEUTRAL.

SERVES 4

Two 3.5 ounce packages angel hair Konjac, Shiratake, or Miracle Noodles
3 tablespoons olive oil
3 cups cubed chicken
Salt to taste
¼ cup chopped olives
¼ cup chopped parsley
3 garlic cloves, minced
4 cups baby spinach
2 cups halved cherry tomatoes
1 cup chicken broth
½ cup white wine
1 teaspoon dried basil
Salt and pepper to taste

1. Rinse the pasta in a colander with cold water for 2 minutes. Dry thoroughly with paper towels, and set aside.
2. Heat the oil in a large fry pan over medium-high heat. Add the chicken, and cook, stirring occasionally, until done, about 10 to 12 minutes.
3. Remove the chicken, and add the remaining ingredients to the pan. Cover and cook over medium heat for about 15 minutes.
4. Stir in the chicken, and serve over the pasta.

Philly Cheese Steak

For Steps One, Two, and Three;

5-GRAM COUNTER CARB OR 11- TO 20-GRAM CARB DAM.

SERVES 4

---

1 pound "minute"/wafer steaks or very thinly sliced skirt or flank steaks (beef or chicken)

2 green bell peppers, cored and sliced into 1-inch strips

1 large onion, diced

2 garlic cloves, finely chopped

½ cup beef or chicken broth

1 cup shredded provolone cheese

1. Preheat the oven to 350°F. Spray a large skillet and a shallow baking pan with cooking spray.
2. Break the wafer steaks into quarters, place in the skillet, and quickly brown. Drain off the excess fat, and place the browned steak quarters in the baking pan.
3. Sauté in the hot skillet over medium-high heat the bell peppers, onion, and garlic until golden brown. Spoon the vegetables on top of the steak.
4. Pour the broth over the steak and veggies, and bake, uncovered, for 20 minutes.
5. Top with the cheese, and broil for 3 minutes, until the cheese begins to bubble.

For Step One, serve inside a low-carb wrap (5 or fewer grams of net carb) to make a 5-gram Counter Carb.

For Steps Two and Three, serve in a warm, 11- to 20-gram net carb bun to make an 11- to 20-gram Carb Dam or one carb serving.

Seafood Delight

For Steps One, Two, and Three; COUNT AS NEUTRAL.

SERVES 4 TO 6

¼ cup butter

¼ cup olive oil

¼ cup white wine

2 teaspoons crushed garlic

½ pound flounder filet

1 pound sea scallops

1 pound whole, cleaned, and deveined shrimp

2 tablespoons finely chopped fresh parsley

¼ cup grated Parmesan cheese

1. Preheat the oven to 400°F. Spray a glass baking dish with cooking spray.
2. Melt the butter in a small saucepan over medium heat, then add the oil, wine, and garlic. Heat until the garlic is lightly browned, then remove and discard the garlic. Set the sauce aside.
3. Cut the flounder into six pieces, and arrange the flounder, scallops, and shrimp in the baking dish.
4. Pour the sauce over the fish, and sprinkle with the parsley. Bake, uncovered, until the fish is flaky and thoroughly cooked.
5. Sprinkle with the Parmesan, if desired, and serve.

Cold Salmon, Quinoa, and Asparagus Salad

For Steps Two and Three; 11- TO 20-GRAM CARB DAM, OR ONE CARB SERVING.

SERVES 4

---

4 cups reduced-sodium chicken broth

1 pound asparagus, cut into 3-inch pieces

1 cup rinsed quinoa

Four 5-ounce salmon filets

Salt and pepper to taste

1 cup feta cheese

2 teaspoons dill weed

2 tablespoons lemon juice

2 tablespoons olive oil

1. Preheat the broiler (or toaster oven broiler).
2. Bring chicken broth to a boil in a medium saucepan over medium-high heat. Add the asparagus and quinoa, and cook for about 4 minutes. Remove the asparagus, and continue cooking the quinoa, stirring occasionally, until it is soft, about 20 minutes. Transfer to a large mixing bowl to cool.
3. While the quinoa is cooking, season the salmon with salt and pepper, and broil for 7 minutes, or until it is opaque throughout. Allow to cool, then flake the salmon into a bowl, cover, and refrigerate for least 1 hour.
4. Whisk together in a separate bowl the feta, dill, lemon juice, oil, and pepper to taste, and add to the quinoa. Add the asparagus, and mix it all together.
5. When ready to serve, toss the salad again, divide onto plates, and top each salad with salmon.

Breaded Baked Flounder

For Steps One, Two, and Three; 5-GRAM COUNTER CARB.

SERVES 4

1.5 pounds flounder

½ teaspoon paprika

½ plus ⅛ teaspoon salt

4 slices low-carb bread, well toasted or left out overnight to dry

4 eggs

1 teaspoon dill

1 teaspoon garlic powder

1. Preheat the oven to 400°F. Line a baking sheet with parchment paper and coat with cooking spray.

2. Season the flounder with the paprika and ⅛ teaspoon of the salt.

3. Place the toast in a food processor, and pulse to make bread crumbs. Transfer to a dinner-sized plate.

4. Whisk together in a small mixing bowl the eggs, ½ teaspoon salt, dill, and garlic powder.

5. Bread the flounder by dipping both sides into the egg mixture, and then dipping each side into the breadcrumbs.

6. Place the flounder on the baking sheet, lightly spray with cooking spray, and bake for about 10 minutes, or until opaque throughout.

Shish Kebab

For Steps One, Two, and Three; COUNT AS NEUTRAL.

SERVES 4 TO 6

¼ cup olive oil

½ cup Italian dressing

2 tablespoons lemon juice

3 large garlic cloves, crushed

¼ cup white wine

¼ teaspoon salt

¼ teaspoon pepper

¼ teaspoon dried oregano

¼ teaspoon dried rosemary

1½ pounds leg of lamb or London broil, cubed for kebabs

1 large green bell pepper, seeded and cut into 8 chunks

1 large red bell pepper, seeded and cut into 8 chunks

1 large red onion, cut into 8 chunks

12 medium mushroom caps

1. Combine in a medium mixing bowl the oil, Italian dressing, lemon juice, garlic, wine, and seasonings. Pour the marinade over the lamb, and stir to coat completely. Cover tightly, and refrigerate for 24 hours, occasionally stirring the sauce over the lamb.

2. The next day, preheat the broiler.

3. Remove the lamb cubes from the marinade, reserving the marinade, and thread them onto skewers to contain only the lamb. Thread other

skewers with the bell peppers, others with the onions, and others with the mushrooms (they will all need different grilling times.)

4. Place the kebabs on a broiling tray, and baste them all with the marinade. Broil about 6 inches from the heat source: the mushroom skewers for 3 minutes, the pepper and the onion skewers for 4 minutes, and the lamb skewers for 10 minutes. Set aside to cool enough to be handled. Unthread all of the lamb and vegetables.

5. Rethread a skewer with a cube of cooked lamb, then a piece of pepper, then onion, and then mushroom, repeating until all ingredients have been used on as many skewers as will hold them.

6. Baste all of the kebabs with the marinade again, and return the skewers to the broiler, turning frequently, until the meat is totally cooked.

Safety note: Because the marinade has been used for raw meat, be sure to cook through at high heat before serving.

Neutral Pizza with Cream Cheese Crust

Steps One, Two, Three; COUNT AS NEUTRAL.

SERVES 4

FOR CRUST

½ cup cream cheese

4 eggs, beaten

⅓ cup half-and-half or light cream

½ cup grated fresh Parmesan cheese

1 teaspoon Italian seasoning

1 teaspoon garlic powder

¾ teaspoon salt

½ teaspoon black pepper

2 cups shredded part-skim mozzarella cheese

FOR SAUCE

¾ cup marinara sauce (no sugar added—only tomatoes, herbs, and spices)

½ teaspoon Italian seasoning

½ teaspoon garlic powder

¼ teaspoon black pepper
¼ teaspoon oregano

FOR TOPPINGS

1½ cups shredded mozzarella cheese
Other popular toppings, such as onions, bell peppers, sausage
  crumbles, mushrooms—add your own favorites!

1. Preheat the oven to 375°F. Lightly spray a round pizza-type baking
   pan with cooking spray; set aside.
2. Whip together in a large bowl the cream cheese and eggs until smooth.
   Add half-and-half, Parmesan, Italian seasoning, garlic powder, salt,
   and pepper; mix well and set aside.
3. Sprinkle 2 cups of the mozzarella evenly in the bottom of the pizza
   baking pan, and bake for 5 minutes. Remove from the oven, and spoon
   the cream cheese mixture over the mozzarella. This will become the
   pizza's "crust." Bake the crust for 30 minutes, and remove from oven.
4. While the crust is baking, simmer the marinara, Italian seasoning,
   garlic powder, pepper, and oregano.
5. Spread the crust with the marinara and 1½ cups of the mozzarella
   and any toppings you prefer!
6. Bake about 12 minutes, or until bubbly. Wait 5 minutes after removing from the oven, then cut into 8 slices.

Swedish Meatballs

For Steps One, Two, and Three; COUNT AS NEUTRAL.

SERVES 4

---

1 pound lean ground beef
1 medium onion, finely chopped
1 medium green bell pepper, seeded and finely chopped
2 garlic cloves, finely chopped
¼ cup finely chopped fresh dill
¼ cup finely chopped fresh parsley
½ teaspoon Italian seasoning

¼ teaspoon grated nutmeg

1 teaspoon dried dill

1 large egg, beaten

½ teaspoon salt

Black pepper to taste

2 tablespoons olive oil

¾ cup beef broth

¼ cup white wine

1. Combine in a large mixing bowl the beef, onion, bell pepper, garlic, dill, parsley, spices, egg, salt, and pepper. Using plastic gloves, use your hands to mix the ingredients evenly. Form into about thirty 1-inch mini-meatballs.

2. Spray a nonstick skillet with cooking spray, and heat the oil over medium heat. Cook the meatballs, in batches if necessary, shaking the skillet occasionally until they are browned on all sides and cooked through. Remove the meatballs from the skillet, and place them on paper towels to drain the excess grease.

3. Add the broth and wine to the skillet, and cover. Increase the heat to high, and cook for about 3 minutes. Add the meatballs back to the pan, and cook in the sauce for 10 minutes, spooning the sauce over the meatballs as it thickens. Serve immediately.

Crockpot Chili

For Step One, you can substitute 2 cans black or white soy beans in place of the kidney and chickpeas for a Neutral chili!

For Steps Two and Three; 11- TO 20-GRAM CARB DAM, OR ONE CARB SERVING.

SERVES 8

One 14-ounce can diced tomatoes, undrained

One 14-ounce can chopped tomatoes and green chili peppers, undrained

1 cup vegetable juice cocktail or low-sodium tomato juice

1 cup low-sodium beef broth

1 tablespoon chili powder

1 teaspoon ground cumin

1 teaspoon dried oregano

3 garlic cloves, peeled and minced

2 pounds boneless beef chuck roast, cut into 1-inch cubes

2 large onions, chopped

3 stalks celery, chopped

1 large green bell pepper, seeded and chopped

One 15-ounce can kidney beans, drained

One 15-ounce can chickpeas (garbanzo beans), drained

(For Step One use 2 cans black or white soy beans in place of kidney
    beans and chickpeas)

1. Place in a 6-quart slow cooker all of the tomatoes, the vegetable juice,
   broth, chili powder, cumin, oregano, garlic, beef, onion, celery, and
   bell peppers. Cover and cook on LOW for 8 to 10 hours or HIGH for 4 to
   5 hours.
2. Stir in the kidney beans and chickpeas (or soy beans for Step One),
   then cook on the HIGH setting for 15 minutes longer.

Eggplant Rollatini

For Steps One, Two, and Three; COUNT AS NEUTRAL.

SERVES 6

---

3 medium eggplants, cut lengthwise into ¼-inch slices

Salt

Olive oil

2 cups part-skim ricotta cheese

1 large egg, beaten

1 cup shredded mozzarella cheese

½ cup grated Parmesan cheese, plus more for topping, optional

¼ cup finely chopped fresh parsley

2 cups seasoned crushed tomatoes or your own marinara sauce, made
    without added tomato paste or tomato sauce

1. Preheat the oven to 350°F. Coat a glass baking dish with cooking spray.

2. Lightly sprinkle both sides of the eggplant with salt. Place the eggplant in a colander in the sink for about 15 minutes, then rinse and blot dry.

3. Heat a large sauté pan sprayed with cooking spray over medium heat. Add 2 tablespoons of olive oil. Add the eggplant in batches, and cook until it is soft and pliable, replacing the olive oil as needed. Transfer the cooked eggplant to a platter.

4. Mix in a large mixing bowl the ricotta, egg, mozzarella, Parmesan, and parsley.

5. Take one eggplant slice, spread a small amount of the cheese mixture over it, and then roll it up. Place the roll, seam side down, into the baking dish. Repeat for the remaining eggplant slices.

6. After all of the eggplant is rolled, pour the tomatoes over the rolls, and top with a little more Parmesan, if desired. Bake for 30 minutes and serve.

All-Veggie Lasagna

For Steps One, Two, and Three; COUNT AS NEUTRAL.

SERVES 9

---

1 large or two small eggplants, cut lengthwise into ½-inch slices

2 pounds part-skim ricotta cheese

4 garlic cloves, chopped

¼ cup grated Parmesan cheese

2 cups shredded part-skim mozzarella

1 bunch fresh basil, chopped

1 tablespoon Italian seasoning

Salt and pepper to taste

1 small onion, chopped

1 medium red, yellow, or orange bell pepper, seeded and chopped

4 cups sliced mushrooms

1 bunch broccoli, florets only, coarsely chopped

3 ounces fresh spinach, chopped

2 cups crushed tomatoes or marinara sauce (jarred or your own with no added tomato paste or tomato sauce)

3 small zucchini, cut lengthwise into ⅛-inch slices

3 small yellow squash, cut lengthwise into ⅛-inch slices

1. Preheat the oven to 350°F. Spray a baking sheet with cooking spray.
2. Arrange the eggplant slices on the baking sheet, and bake for 15 to 20 minutes, until flexible but not completely cooked.
3. Mix in a bowl the ricotta with half of the garlic. Stir in the Parmesan and 1½ cups of the mozzarella, the basil, Italian seasoning, and salt and pepper, and set aside.
4. Sauté the onion, remaining garlic, bell pepper, mushrooms, and broccoli for about 5 minutes. Add the spinach, and remove from the heat. Allow to cool, and then add to the ricotta mixture.
5. To assemble, spread a thin layer of the tomatoes in a large baking dish, such as a 3-quart Pyrex lasagna dish, then layer:
   eggplant slices
   ricotta mixture
   zucchini or squash slices
   tomatoes
6. Repeat the layering until you run out of ingredients. End with a layer of zucchini or eggplant, and top with tomatoes. Sprinkle with the reserved ½ cup of mozzarella.
7. Bake for 1 to 1½ hours, until hot and bubbly.

Turkey Frittata

For Steps One, Two, and Three; COUNT AS NEUTRAL.

SERVES 4

¼ cup olive oil

½ pound ground lean turkey

1 sweet onion, finely chopped

1 green bell pepper, finely chopped

1 teaspoon minced garlic

6 large eggs

1 teaspoon hot sauce

½ cup unsweetened soy or almond milk

Salt and pepper to taste

1. Preheat the oven to 425°F.
2. Heat the oil in a large "stove to oven" fry pan over medium-high heat. Add the turkey, onion, bell pepper, and garlic, and sauté, breaking apart the turkey with a fork as the turkey cooks. Cook until the turkey is no longer pink, about 12 minutes. Drain the turkey in a colander to remove the grease, and return it to the fry pan.
3. Whisk together in a medium mixing bowl the eggs, hot sauce, milk, and salt and pepper to taste. Pour over the ground turkey, lower the heat to medium, and cook, without stirring, 2 to 3 minutes, or until the eggs begin to set.
4. Transfer the fry pan to the oven, and bake for about 5 minutes.

Open-Faced Portobello Cap Sandwich

For Steps One, Two, and Three; 5-GRAM COUNTER CARB.

SERVES 1

---

1 teaspoon minced garlic
2 teaspoons balsamic vinegar
1 tablespoon olive oil
1 teaspoon Classic Pesto (page 279)
1 portobello mushroom cap, cleaned and gills removed
2 teaspoons light mayonnaise
1 slice toasted low-carb bread (5 or fewer grams net carb)
Leaf of Romaine lettuce
2 fresh tomato slices

1. Preheat the grill to medium-high. Coat a sheet of aluminum foil with cooking spray.
2. Whisk together in a small bowl the garlic, vinegar, oil, and pesto.
3. Place the mushroom on the foil, drizzle half of the sauce over the mushroom, and place on the hot grill. Grill for 3 to 4 minutes per side, covered.
4. Combine the remaining sauce with the mayonnaise, and spread it on the toast. Top with the lettuce and tomato, then finish with the grilled mushroom cap.

Stuffed Peppers

For Steps Two and Three; 11- TO 20-GRAM CARB DAM, OR ONE CARB SERVING.

SERVES 4

---

4 medium green bell peppers
½ cup sugar-free ketchup
1 teaspoon Worcestershire sauce
½ pound ground lean turkey
1 cup cooked brown rice
1 large egg, beaten
1 cup frozen corn
1 teaspoon salt
¼ teaspoon pepper

1. Preheat the oven to 350°F. Coat a baking dish with cooking spray.
2. Wash the peppers, cut the tops off (reserve the tops), core and remove the seeds, and set aside.
3. Whisk together in a small mixing bowl the ketchup, 1 cup of water, and the Worcestershire sauce, and set aside.
4. Mix together in a large mixing bowl the turkey, rice, egg, corn, salt, and pepper.
5. Put ¼ of the turkey mixture into each pepper, then replace the top of each pepper.
6. Place the filled peppers in the baking dish, pour the ketchup mixture over the stuffed peppers, and bake for 45 minutes.

Side Dishes

Low-Carb Cranberry Sauce

For Steps One, Two, and Three; COUNT AS 5-GRAM COUNTER CARB.

SERVES 4

---

1 cup Splenda or Swerve
One 12-ounce package fresh cranberries
Whipped cream

1. Combine the Splenda with 1 cup of water in a medium saucepan; bring to a boil. Add the cranberries; return to a boil. Reduce heat, and boil gently for 10 minutes, stirring occasionally. Cover, remove from the stove, and cool completely to room temperature.
2. Refrigerate until serving time, and serve chilled. Add a dollop of whipped cream for an extra pop.

Broccoli-Cheese Casserole

For Steps One, Two, and Three; COUNT AS NEUTRAL.

SERVES 4

---

2 cups shredded Cheddar cheese
2 cups sliced mushrooms
1 cup chopped scallions
½ cup light cream
¼ cup olive oil
½ teaspoon salt
2 cups chopped fresh broccoli

1. Preheat the oven to 350°F. Coat a 2-quart casserole dish with cooking spray.
2. Combine all of the ingredients in a medium saucepan, and warm over medium-low heat. Cook for 5 minutes, stirring constantly, until the cheese is melted. Spoon the mixture into the casserole dish, and bake for 30 minutes. Serve warm.

"Faux" Mashed Potatoes

For Steps One, Two, and Three; COUNT AS NEUTRAL.

SERVES 4

---

1 head cauliflower, florets only
2 garlic cloves, finely chopped
½ onion, finely chopped
1 (14-ounce) can chicken broth
½ teaspoon salt
¼ teaspoon pepper
1 tablespoon butter
¼ cup light sour cream
½ cup reduced-fat shredded Cheddar cheese
Salt and pepper to taste

1. Combine the cauliflower, garlic, onion, broth, and salt in a medium saucepan, and heat over medium-high heat; bring to a boil. Reduce the heat to medium, and simmer until the vegetables are extremely tender. Drain, reserving the broth.
2. Transfer the cauliflower mixture to a large mixing bowl, and add the pepper, butter, sour cream, and cheese. Whip the cauliflower mixture with a hand mixer until it is the consistency of whipped potatoes, adding the reserved broth as needed. Salt and pepper to taste. Serve warm as you would mashed potatoes.

Sweet Potato Fries with "Maple Syrup" Dip

For Steps Two and Three; 11- TO 20-GRAMS CARB DAM, OR ONE CARB SERVING.

SERVES 4

2 sweet potatoes, peeled and cut lengthwise in ¼-inch strips
Salt and pepper to taste
1 teaspoon ground cinnamon
Carb-free maple-flavored syrup

1. Preheat the oven to 450°F. Coat a cookie sheet with cooking spray.
2. Arrange the sweet potato strips on the sheet; do not overlap. Spray the potatoes with cooking spray, then sprinkle with salt and pepper.
3. Bake, turning every 10 minutes, for 30 to 45 minutes, or until tender.
4. When done, sprinkle with cinnamon and dip in warm carb-free syrup. Serve warm.

Honeyed Sweet Potato

For Steps Two and Three; 11- TO 20-GRAM CARB DAM, OR ONE CARB SERVING.

SERVES 4

2 sweet potatoes
2 tablespoons olive oil
Salt to taste
4 teaspoons whipped butter
½ cup Greek yogurt
2 teaspoons honey

1. Wash each sweet potato, then use a fork to prick holes into its skin. Coat with oil, and microwave on a paper towel or a microwave-safe plate on HIGH for 10 minutes or until soft.
2. Split the potatoes open lengthwise, and sprinkle each half with salt, then top with butter, Greek yogurt, and honey.
3. Return to the microwave for 30 seconds to heat the topping. Serve immediately.

Tabbouleh

For Steps Two and Three; 11- TO 20-GRAM CARB DAM, OR ONE CARB SERVING.
SERVES 6

---

1 cup uncooked bulgur

2 cups boiling water

⅓ cup lemon juice

½ teaspoon salt

¼ teaspoon black pepper

2 garlic cloves, minced

3 medium tomatoes, seeded and chopped

1 cup finely chopped parsley

1 cup finely chopped scallions

½ cup finely chopped mint leaves

Greek yogurt for garnish

1. Combine the bulgur with the boiling water in a bowl; let soak for 1 hour.
2. Combine in a large mixing bowl the lemon juice, salt, pepper, and garlic.
3. Drain the bulgur, and add it to the lemon juice mixture. Add the remaining ingredients, and mix thoroughly.
4. Cover tightly and refrigerate for at least 1 hour. Serve chilled with a dollop of yogurt.

Miracle Baked Beans

For Steps One, Two, and Three; COUNT AS NEUTRAL.
SERVES 6 TO 8

---

8 slices bacon, chopped

1 medium onion, chopped

¾ cup reduced-sugar ketchup

¾ cup canned tomatoes, pureed

½ cup granular Splenda

¼ cup apple cider vinegar or red wine vinegar

1 tablespoon Worcestershire sauce

Salt and pepper to taste

Four 15-ounce cans of black soy beans, drained and rinsed (can mix black soy beans and regular soy beans)

1. Preheat oven to 350°F.
2. Heat a Dutch oven (or heavy-bottomed pot with a lid that can go in the oven) over medium-high heat. Add the bacon and cook, stirring often, until the fat renders and the bacon begins to crisp, about 6 to 8 minutes. Add the onion, and cook until it is softened, about 5 minutes more. Stir in the ketchup, tomatoes, Splenda, vinegar, Worcestershire, and salt and pepper, and mix well. Bring to a simmer, and cook for 5 minutes.
3. Stir in the beans until they are well coated, cover, and bake for 1 hour. Then remove the lid and continue baking until the sauce thickens and the beans begin to brown, about 15 minutes more. Remove from the oven, and cool for at least 15 minutes before serving. Serve warm.

Cauliflower Rice

For Steps One, Two, and Three; COUNT AS NEUTRAL.

SERVES 4

---

1 head cauliflower

Salt to taste

1. Chop the cauliflower in a food processor or grate with a hand grater until it is the size of rice (use the plain steel or shredder blade in the food processor).
2. Sprinkle the cauliflower with salt, place it in a microwave-safe bowl, cover, and microwave on HIGH for 4 minutes. *Do not add water*—this faux "rice" will fluff up from the cauliflower's moisture.

Cauliflower rice is bland but will absorb the flavor of stir fries or sauces. Use it in place of white rice. You can add butter, Parmesan cheese, and parsley to make it into a side dish.

Sweet Things

Lemon Lime-Ade

For Steps One, Two, Three; COUNT AS NEUTRAL.

SERVES 6

---

4 cups cold water
1 cup lemon juice
½ cup lime juice
1 cup Splenda or the equivalent of stevia or erythritol
2 cups ice

IF USING ICE CUBES

Pour the water, fruit juices, Splenda, and 1 cup of the ice in a blender; blend on HIGH for 1 minute; add the other 1 cup of ice cubes, and blend on HIGH for another minute. Serve.

IF USING CRUSHED ICE

Combine all of the ingredients in a blender; blend on HIGH for 1½ minutes. Serve.

For an even slushier consistency, place in the freezer for about 20 minutes before enjoying!

Peppermint Mocha Coffee Creamer

Steps One, Two, Three; COUNT AS NEUTRAL.

MAKES 16 OUNCES (2 CUPS) CREAMER

---

1 cup half-and-half

1 cup unsweetened vanilla almond milk

5 tablespoons cocoa powder

2 teaspoons pure peppermint extract

5 tablespoons Splenda or stevia

1. Place all of the ingredients in a blender, and blend until everything is smooth and combined.
2. Pour into an airtight container and refrigerate. Shake it up before using!

Holiday Egg Nog

Steps One, Two, Three: COUNT AS NEUTRAL.

SERVES 1

---

2 tablespoons heavy cream (whip for a fluffier egg nog)

¼ cup Egg Beaters (or other double-pasteurized liquid egg substitute)

2 tablespoons Splenda or stevia

½ cup half-and-half or light creamer

½ teaspoon vanilla extract

Nutmeg for garnish

1. Whip the heavy cream until it is fluffy and light.
2. Place the remaining ingredients in a blender; blend on HIGH until the Splenda dissolves. Transfer to a bowl.
3. Right before serving, gently fold in the whipped heavy cream. Sprinkle with nutmeg.

According to the Egg Beaters site, Egg Beaters are double pasteurized and safe to consume uncooked.

Cool and Creamy Jell-O Mousse

For Steps One, Two, and Three; COUNT AS NEUTRAL.

SERVES 8

One 4-serving package sugar-free Jell-O, any flavor
One 8-ounce container light cream cheese, softened
½ cup light sour cream
1 cup light whipping cream
2 teaspoons powdered Splenda

1. Prepare the Jell-O as directed on the box. Refrigerate until it is almost set but still a little soft, about 1 hour 15 minutes.
2. Remove the Jell-O from the refrigerator, and beat with a hand mixer until it is creamy. While continuing to beat with the mixer, add the cream cheese and sour cream, and mix thoroughly.
3. Whip together in a separate bowl the whipping cream and Splenda until peaks form. Gently fold the whipped cream into the gelatin mixture, leaving it with a marbled look—don't keep stirring until it becomes uniform in color.
4. Spoon into dessert dishes, and chill for at least 2 hours before serving.

Breads and Bread Products

Cheddar Cheese Biscuits

For Steps One, Two, Three; COUNT AS NEUTRAL.

SERVES 8

2½ cups blanched almond flour

1 cup shredded low-fat Cheddar cheese

½ teaspoon salt

½ teaspoon baking soda

¼ teaspoon garlic powder

¼ teaspoon onion powder

¼ teaspoon Old Bay seasoning

¼ teaspoon dried rosemary

½ teaspoon dried parsley flakes

½ cup plus 3 tablespoons unsalted butter

4 large eggs, lightly beaten

2 tablespoons grated Parmesan cheese

½ teaspoon parsley flakes

1. Preheat the oven to 350°F. Line a cookie sheet with parchment paper.
2. Stir together in a large bowl the flour, Cheddar, salt, baking soda, garlic powder, onion powder, Old Bay, rosemary, and parsley flakes. Cut in ½ of the butter (cold from the refrigerator), using a fork or pastry blender, until crumbly. Add the eggs, and mix to form a dough. (Use plastic gloves if you are using hands to mix the dough.)
3. Divide the dough (with gloved hands) into 8 portions, and form into balls. Place on the baking tray, and flatten slightly. (Insulated baking trays help prevent burning.) Bake for 15 to 20 minutes, or until an

inserted toothpick in the middle of a biscuit comes out clean. If the baking tray is not insulated, check frequently for timing.

4. Melt 3 tablespoons of the butter with the parsley, and brush on the top of the biscuits while they are still warm. Immediately sprinkle with the Parmesan.

Cheddar Flax Crackers

For Steps One, Two, and Three; COUNT AS NEUTRAL.

SERVES 6

Olive oil cooking spray
1 cup ground flaxseed or flaxseed meal
1 cup shredded Cheddar cheese
1 cup water
Dash of chili powder
Dash of garlic powder
Dash of paprika
Sea salt, for garnish, optional
Sesame seeds, for garnish, optional

1. Preheat the oven to 375°F. Coat a cookie sheet with cooking spray.
2. Combine the remaining ingredients in a medium bowl. Oil your hands to knead the mixture into a firm dough; form it into a ball. Press the dough onto the cookie sheet, making a thin layer. Spray the dough with the olive oil cooking spray, and top with sea salt and sesame seeds, if desired. Bake for 25 minutes.
3. When it begins to cool, use a sharp knife or cooking scissors to cut it into cracker-sized pieces. Let them cool completely, then store in an airtight container.

Light and Airy Dinner Rolls

For Steps One, Two, Three; COUNT AS NEUTRAL.

MAKES 9 TO 12 DINNER ROLLS

3 eggs, separated

1/8 teaspoon cream of tartar

3 ounces light cream cheese, cold, or 3 tablespoons low-fat ricotta or
cottage cheese, cold

1/2 teaspoon Splenda

Pinch of salt

1. Preheat the oven to 300°F. Coat the cups of a muffin tin with cooking spray and set aside.
2. Whip together in a medium bowl the egg whites with the cream of tartar for 3 to 4 minutes or until very stiff peaks form; set aside.
3. Beat together in a large bowl the cream cheese. While still beating, add the egg yolks until smooth. Beat in the Splenda and salt for 2 minutes until the mixture is light yellow.
4. Gently fold 1/3 of the egg whites into the yolk mixture to lighten, then fold in the remaining whites until all fluffs disappear, but be careful not to deflate them.
5. Fill each muffin cup 2/3 full with the mixture, and bake for about 20 minutes, but toward the end check frequently: the rolls should be a deep golden brown.
6. Immediately loosen the muffins, but don't remove, and allow them to cool for a few minutes in the tin. Remove them, and transfer to a wire rack to cool completely. Store in an airtight container or plastic bag.

The Miracle Bun

For Steps One, Two, and Three; COUNT AS NEUTRAL.

SERVES 1

---

1 packet stevia or Splenda
2 tablespoons almond meal
2 tablespoons ground flaxseed
½ teaspoon baking powder
¼ teaspoon Italian seasoning, optional for a seasoned bun
Pinch of salt
1 large egg, beaten
1 teaspoon sesame seeds

1. Mix together in a small bowl the sweetener, almond meal, flaxseed, baking powder, Italian seasoning, if desired, and salt. Add the egg, and stir until smooth.
2. Coat a 10-ounce Pyrex custard cup with cooking spray, and sprinkle sesame seeds on the bottom and sides. Pour the batter into the cup, and top with more sesame seeds.
3. Microwave on HIGH for approximately 90 seconds.
4. Run a butter knife around the side of the cup to loosen the bun, and remove.

Baked Goods

Thumbprint Peanut Butter and Jelly Cookies

Step One, Two, and Three; 3 COOKIES = 5-GRAM COUNTER CARB.

MAKES ABOUT 18 COOKIES

¼ teaspoon salt

½ teaspoon baking soda

1 egg or ¼ cup Egg Beaters or 2 egg whites

½ teaspoon vanilla extract

¼ cup erythritol (Swerve)

1 teaspoon stevia powder

1 cup natural peanut butter (no added sugar, just peanuts, salt, and oil)

¼ cup unsweetened applesauce

Polaner or Smucker's sugar-free jelly (any flavor)

1. Preheat the oven to 350°F. Line a baking sheet with parchment paper.
2. Whisk together in a medium mixing bowl the salt, baking soda, egg, and vanilla. Add in the erythritol and stevia, and mix well. Stir in the peanut butter and applesauce; mix together until it is all combined.
3. The cookie dough will be crumbly. Roll into teaspoon-sized balls, and make a small indentation in the center of each with your pointer finger. Fill the depression of each cookie with about ¼ teaspoon of the jelly. Arrange cookies about 2 inches apart on the baking sheet.
4. Bake for about 11 minutes, until lightly browned. Cool on a baking sheet for two minutes, then transfer to a wire rack to cool.

Baked Apples

For Steps Two and Three; 11- TO 20-GRAM CARB DAM, OR ONE CARB SERVING.

SERVES 4

¼ cup butter, softened

4 tablespoons powdered Splenda

½ teaspoon ground cinnamon

½ teaspoon grated nutmeg

½ teaspoon ground allspice

4 large baking apples (e.g., Empire, Cortland, Golden Delicious, Wine sap), washed and cored

1. Preheat the oven to 350°F. Coat a baking dish with cooking spray and set aside.
2. Blend in a small mixing bowl the butter, Splenda, and spices. Divide evenly four ways, and spoon into the apples.
3. Place the apples in the baking dish, and bake for 30 minutes, or until the apples are tender. Serve warm.

Chocolate Brownie Muffins

For Steps One, Two, and Three; COUNT AS NEUTRAL.

MAKES ABOUT 20 MUFFINS

---

5 ounces unsweetened baking chocolate

2 cups powdered Splenda

¾ cup soy flour

1 cup almond flour

1½ teaspoons baking powder

1½ teaspoons baking soda

1 teaspoon salt

2 eggs

One 16-ounce container light sour cream

½ cup olive oil

2 teaspoons vanilla extract

½ cup finely chopped walnuts, optional
1 cup boiling water

1. Preheat the oven to 350°F. Line 20 to 24 muffin cups with cupcake liners.
2. Microwave the chocolate on HIGH for about 2 minutes, until it is melted. (Cover while microwaving to avoid spattering.)
3. Combine the dry ingredients in a mixing bowl. Add the eggs, melted chocolate, sour cream, oil, and vanilla. Stir in the nuts, if desired. Slowly pour in the boiling water while mixing to a smooth batter. The batter will be thin.
4. Fill each muffin cup ⅔ full, and bake for 22 to 25 minutes. Cool on cooling rack.

These muffins are great for freezing in freezer bags and pulling out as needed. They can be topped with light whipped cream.

Cinnamon Muffins

For Step One, Two, and Three; COUNT AS NEUTRAL.

MAKES ABOUT 20 MUFFINS

2 cups soy flour
2 cups almond flour
1½ teaspoons baking soda
1½ teaspoons baking powder
1 teaspoon salt
4 teaspoons ground cinnamon
4 eggs
½ cup oil
1½ cups Splenda
One 16-ounce container light sour cream

1. Preheat the oven to 350°F. Coat 24 muffin cups with cooking spray or line with cupcake liners.
2. Mix together in a large mixing bowl the flours, baking soda, baking powder, salt, and cinnamon.

3. Beat together in a separate bowl the eggs, and blend with the oil and Splenda. Mix for about 30 seconds.
4. Combine the egg mixture with the dry mixture, and then blend in the sour cream.
5. Pour the batter into the muffin cups, and bake for 25 minutes, or until lightly browned. Cool on a cooling rack.

Zucchini Muffins

For Steps One, Two, and Three; COUNT AS NEUTRAL.
MAKES 20 TO 24 MUFFINS

2 cups soy flour
1 2/3 cups almond flour
1/3 cup ground flaxseed
1½ teaspoons baking soda
1½ teaspoons baking powder
1 teaspoon salt
1½ teaspoons ground cinnamon
4 eggs
½ cup oil
1¼ cups Splenda
2 medium zucchinis, shredded (about 2 cups)
1 cup light sour cream
1 cup walnut pieces, optional

1. Preheat the oven to 350°F. Coat 24 muffin cups with cooking spray or line with cupcake liners.
2. Whisk together in a large bowl the flours, flaxseed, baking soda, baking powder, salt, and cinnamon.
3. Mix in a separate bowl the eggs, oil, and Splenda for 30 seconds, until the sugar substitute is dissolved. Stir in the zucchini.
4. Stir the egg mixture into the flour mixture. Stir in the sour cream and then the walnuts, if using.
5. Pour the batter into the muffin cups, filling them 2/3 full. If all 24 cups will not be used, fill each of the empty cups with a few tablespoons of water.

6. Bake for 23 to 25 minutes, or until crowned and lightly browned. Cool on a cooling rack.

Carrot Cake with Cream Cheese Frosting

For Steps One, Two, Three; 5-GRAM COUNTER CARB.

MAKES 12 SLICES OF CAKE

---

4 cups almond flour

1½ cups Splenda

½ cup erythritol (Swerve)

2 teaspoons baking soda

2 teaspoons baking powder

½ teaspoon salt

1 tablespoon ground cinnamon

½ teaspoon ground ginger

¼ teaspoon ground nutmeg

4 eggs

¼ cup oil

½ cup sour cream

1 tablespoon vanilla extract

3 cups grated carrots

1 cup chopped pecans

Neutral Cream Cheese Frosting (page 334)

1. Preheat the oven to 350°F. Spray a 9 × 13-inch cake pan with cooking spray.
2. Combine in a large mixing bowl the dry ingredients, and stir well.
3. Beat the eggs, oil, sour cream, and vanilla in a medium mixing bowl until smooth. Add this mixture to the dry ingredients, and mix well. Stir in the carrots and pecans.
4. Pour the batter into the pan, and bake for 40 minutes, or until a toothpick inserted into the middle comes out clean and the cake is firm to the touch. Remove from the oven to a wire rack, and cool completely before spreading the frosting.

Neutral Cream Cheese Frosting

For Steps One, Two, and Three; COUNT AS NEUTRAL.

ICES ONE 9 X 13-INCH CAKE

---

8 ounces low-fat cream cheese, softened

¾ cup powdered Splenda

1 teaspoon vanilla extract

Beat together all of the ingredients in a medium mixing bowl until smooth.

To make powdered Splenda: Combine ¾ cup Splenda with 2 tablespoons cornstarch in a food processor or blender; process until Splenda is a very fine powder.

Pumpkin Spice Muffins

For Steps One, Two, Three; ONE MUFFIN = 5-GRAM COUNTER CARB

MAKES 10 TO 12 MUFFINS

1½ cups almond flour

1 tablespoon pumpkin pie spice

⅔ cup erythritol (Swerve) sweetener

⅔ cup canned plain pumpkin

4 extra-large eggs or 1 cup egg substitute

1 teaspoon vanilla extract

½ cup chopped walnuts, optional

1. Preheat the oven to 300°F. Line 10 to 12 muffin cups with cupcake liners.
2. Combine the dry ingredients in a large bowl, and mix well.
3. Add the pumpkin, eggs, and vanilla, and beat with a mixer until the batter is smooth. Stir in the walnuts, if desired, until they are evenly distributed.
4. Scoop the batter evenly into the muffin cups, and bake for 30 to 40 minutes, or until a toothpick inserted into the middle of a muffin comes out almost dry. Muffin tops will be golden in color.

5. Remove the muffin pan from the oven, and place it on a cooling rack; cover the muffins with a clean towel to trap moisture while they cool.
6. When the muffins have cooled, store in an airtight container. The muffins may be frozen for future use.

Cinnamon Ricotta Pudding

For Steps One, Two, and Three; COUNT AS NEUTRAL.

SERVES 1

½ cup part-skim ricotta cheese
1 tablespoon low-fat sour cream
¼ teaspoon vanilla extract
¼ teaspoon ground cinnamon
1 packet Splenda or stevia
Light whipped cream

1. Mix together in a dessert bowl the ricotta, sour cream, vanilla, cinnamon, and Splenda.
2. Top with the whipped cream before serving. Store in refrigerator.

Chocolate Ricotta Pudding

For Steps One, Two, and Three; COUNT AS NEUTRAL.

SERVES 1

½ cup part-skim ricotta cheese
1 tablespoon low-fat sour cream
½ teaspoon unsweetened cocoa powder
¼ teaspoon vanilla extract
1 packet Splenda
Light whipped cream

1. Mix together in a dessert bowl the ricotta, sour cream, cocoa, vanilla, and Splenda.
2. Top with the whipped cream before serving. Store in refrigerator.

Lemon Ricotta Pudding

For Steps One, Two, and Three; COUNT AS NEUTRAL.

SERVES 1

½ cup part-skim ricotta cheese

1 tablespoon low-fat sour cream

¼ teaspoon grated lemon zest

¼ teaspoon vanilla extract

One 1-gram packet Splenda

Light whipped cream

1. Mix together in a dessert bowl the ricotta, sour cream, zest, vanilla, and Splenda.
2. Top with the whipped cream before serving. Store in refrigerator.

Easy Snickerdoodles

For Steps One, Two, Three; COUNT AS NEUTRAL.

MAKES ABOUT 18 COOKIES

½ cup softened butter

1½ cups almond flour

1¼ cup Splenda or sucralose

1 extra-large egg

1 teaspoon vanilla extract

¼ teaspoon baking soda

¼ teaspoon cream of tartar

2 teaspoons ground cinnamon

1. Preheat the oven to 350°F.
2. Beat the butter in a medium mixing bowl for 30 seconds. Add half of the almond flour, ½ cup of the Splenda, the egg, vanilla, baking soda, and cream of tartar, and beat together until well blended. Then beat in the remaining almond flour and ½ cup of Splenda, and mix well.
3. Cover the mixing bowl, place in the refrigerator, and chill for at least 1 hour.

4. Mix in a small saucer the cinnamon with the remaining ¼ cup of Splenda; set aside.

5. Shape the chilled dough into walnut-sized balls, and roll in the cinnamon mixture until all sides are coated. Place the cookie balls on a cookie sheet about 2 inches apart. Using the bottom of a drinking glass, slightly flatten each cookie ball.

6. Bake for 12 to 14 minutes, or until the bottoms are golden in color. Cool completely before eating. These cookies store best in a freezer bag in the freezer.

Cranberry Walnut Cookies

For Steps One, Two, and Three; COUNT AS NEUTRAL.

MAKES ABOUT 30 COOKIES

½ cup butter, softened

½ cup cream cheese, softened

1½ cups Splenda or Swerve

1 teaspoon vanilla extract

1 teaspoon cinnamon

2 eggs

1½ cups almond meal or almond flour

1 cup low-carb whey protein powder

½ teaspoon baking powder

½ teaspoon baking soda

1 teaspoon salt

¾ cup chopped walnuts

1 cup whole, raw cranberries (fresh or frozen)

1. Preheat the oven to 375°F.

2. Cream the butter and cream cheese in a large mixing bowl until fluffy. Add the Splenda, vanilla, and cinnamon, and beat again. Add the eggs, and beat until the mixture is combined.

3. Combine the almond meal, protein powder, baking powder, baking soda, and salt in a separate bowl, then add the dry mixture to the wet mixture, and beat until it is all combined. Stir in the chopped walnuts and cranberries until they are distributed evenly.

4. Form the batter into rounded spoonfuls, and drop each about 2 inches apart onto an ungreased cookie sheet. Bake about 7 to 9 minutes, until the tops are just browning.
5. Cool completely before eating. Store in a sealed container. The cookies may be frozen for future use.

This recipe also makes for a delicious chocolate-chip cookie. Simply replace the 1 cup of cranberries with ¾ cup of Lily's sugar-free dark chocolate chips. Two to three cookies can count as a 5-gram Counter Carb. After about 4 to 5 minutes of baking, use a fork to flatten down the cookies or they will be too fluffy! This came from Miracle-Ville.com, and members swear by them!

Chocolate Meringues

For Steps One, Two, or Three; 2 TO 3 COOKIES COUNT AS NEUTRAL.
MAKES ABOUT 26 COOKIES

5 egg whites
¼ teaspoon vinegar
1½ teaspoons vanilla extract
½ cup Splenda
¼ cup Splenda Sugar Blend for Baking
¼ cup unsweetened cocoa powder
¼ cup ground pecans, optional

1. Preheat the oven to 200°F. Line several cookie sheets with parchment paper.
2. Whip in a large mixing bowl the egg whites, vinegar, and vanilla extract until they are frothy. Add the Splendas a little at a time; beat until stiff. Gently fold in the cocoa powder and pecans, if using.
3. Using a tablespoon, place spoonfuls of the mixture 1 inch apart onto the cookie sheets. Bake for 1 hour and 30 minutes, then shut off the oven and let the meringues dry for 2 to 3 hours more in the oven. When dried, they will be hardened, light, and airy.
4. Let cool completely, then peel the cookies gently from the parchment. Store in an airtight container.

Chocolate-Dipped Chocolate Meringue Cookies

For Steps One, Two, or Three;

2 TO 3 COOKIES COUNT AS A 5-GRAM COUNTER CARB.

MAKES ABOUT 26 COOKIES

FOR THE MERINGUE

4 large egg whites

¼ teaspoon cream of tartar

½ cup Splenda

2 tablespoons unsweetened cocoa powder

½ teaspoon pure vanilla extract

FOR THE CHOCOLATE COATING

3½ ounces dark chocolate

1½ tablespoons butter

1. Preheat the oven to 200°F. Line two baking sheets with parchment paper.
2. Beat on medium speed in a large mixing bowl the egg whites and cream of tartar. Add the Splenda and cocoa powder, and increase the speed to high until the egg whites form very stiff peaks. Add the vanilla, and mix to incorporate.
3. With a large, star-shaped pastry tip, pipe a 2-inch disc onto the parchment paper, and then pipe another layer on top to form a small peak. Repeat with the remaining meringue batter.
4. Bake for 1 hour and 20 minutes, then turn off the oven and let sit in the oven for 3 hours or until the meringues have dried out.
5. Melt the chocolate and butter in a double boiler and mix well.
6. Dip each meringue cookie into the chocolate (either just the bottom or half of the cookie), and set on parchment paper. Refrigerate until the chocolate has set.

Miracle-Ville's Favorite Neutral Chocolate Cake

For Steps One, Two, or Three; COUNT AS NEUTRAL.

SERVES 9

½ cup butter

¼ cup Hood reduced-carb chocolate milk or unsweetened chocolate almond milk

2 tablespoons unsweetened cocoa powder

3 eggs, beaten or ¾ cup egg substitute

½ cup flaxseed meal

½ cup almond flour

1½ cups Splenda or sucralose

¼ cup light sour cream

1 tablespoon vanilla extract

1 tablespoon ground cinnamon, optional

½ teaspoon baking soda

½ teaspoon baking powder

½ cup chopped nuts, optional

Light whipped cream

1. Preheat the oven to 350°F. Coat an 8-inch-square baking dish with cooking spray.
2. Melt the butter gently in a medium saucepan; add the chocolate milk, then stir in the cocoa. Increase the heat to medium-high, and continue cooking until it is just boiling, stirring constantly to blend well. Remove the saucepan from the stove.
3. Gradually add all of the remaining ingredients into the saucepan, stirring as you go.
4. Pour the mixture into the baking dish, and bake for 25 minutes.
5. Let cool at least 20 minutes. Cut into 9 pieces. Garnish each slice with a dollop of whipped cream.

Appendix

Weight- and Inch-Loss Expectations
on Steps One and Two

There are separate Expected Weight and Inch Loss charts for men and women.

Weigh and measure at the beginning of every eight-week period plus time added for slip-ups. Find your height and weight on the appropriate gender chart to find your expected fat and inch loss at the end of the eight-week period plus time added for slip-ups.

Steps One and Two of the Metabolism Miracle promote muscle retention, fluid balance, and fat burning. As a result of MM's design, you will appear to weigh about ten or more pounds less than your scale weight indicates. For instance, if you lose fifteen pounds (and thirteen to seventeen inches) on MM, it will appear as if you've lost twenty-five.

Women

In the following table, the "weight at start of 8 weeks" is your weight either before starting MM or before starting Step Two. The expected loss column, then, is how much you can expect to lose in pounds and inches either at the end of Step One and before beginning Step Two or at the end of Step Two, respectively.

Women: Expected Fat and Inch Loss after Eight Weeks Plus Time Added for Slip-Ups on Steps One and Two

Height	Weight at start of 8 weeks (pounds)	Expected fat loss in pounds/inches after 8 weeks plus slip-ups	Height	Weight at start of 8 weeks (pounds)	Expected fat loss in pounds/inches after 8 weeks plus slip-ups
4'10"	90 to 130	3 to 5	5'6"	130 to 170	3 to 5
	130 to 170	6 to 13		170 to 210	6 to 13
	170 to 210	14 to 21		210 to 250	14 to 21
	210 to 250	22 to 29		250 to 290	22 to 29
4'11"	95 to 135	3 to 5	5'7"	135 to 175	3 to 5
	135 to 175	6 to 13		175 to 215	6 to 13
	175 to 215	14 to 21		215 to 255	14 to 21
	215 to 255	22 to 29		255 to 295	22 to 29
5'0"	100 to 140	3 to 5	5'8"	140 to 180	3 to 5
	140 to 180	6 to 13		180 to 220	6 to 13
	180 to 220	14 to 21		220 to 260	14 to 21
	220 to 260	22 to 29		260 to 300	22 to 29
5'1"	105 to 145	3 to 5	5'9"	145 to 185	3 to 5
	145 to 185	6 to 13		186 to 225	6 to 13
	185 to 225	14 to 21		225 to 265	14 to 21
	225 to 265	22 to 29		265 to 305	22 to 29
5'2"	110 to 150	3 to 5	5'10"	150 to 190	3 to 5
	150 to 190	6 to 13		190 to 230	6 to 13
	190 to 230	14 to 21		230 to 270	14 to 21
	230 to 270	22 to 29		270 to 310	22 to 29
5'3"	115 to 155	3 to 5	5'11"	155 to 195	3 to 5
	155 to 195	6 to 13		195 to 235	6 to 13
	195 to 235	14 to 21		235 to 275	14 to 21
	235 to 275	22 to 29		275 to 315	22 to 29
5'4"	120 to 160	3 to 5	6'0"	160 to 200	3 to 5
	160 to 200	6 to 13		200 to 240	6 to 13
	200 to 240	14 to 21		240 to 280	14 to 21
	240 to 280	22 to 29		280 to 320	22 to 29
5'5"	125 to 165	3 to 5			
	165 to 205	6 to 13			
	205 to 245	14 to 21			
	245 to 285	22 to 20			

Men

In the following table, the "weight at start of 8 weeks" is your weight either before starting MM or before starting Step Two. The expected loss column, then, is how much you can expect to lose in pounds and inches either at the end of Step One and before beginning Step Two or at the end of Step Two, respectively.

Men: Expected Fat and Inch Loss after Eight Weeks Plus Time Added for Slip-Ups on Steps One and Two

Height	Weight at start of 8 weeks	Expected fat loss in pounds/inches after 8 weeks plus slip-ups	Height	Weight at start of 8 weeks	Expected fat loss in pounds/inches after 8 weeks plus slip-ups
5'0"	106 to 146	3 to 5	5'6"	142 to 182	3 to 5
	146 to 186	6 to 13		182 to 222	6 to 13
	186 to 226	14 to 21		222 to 262	14 to 21
	226 to 266	22 to 29		262 to 302	22 to 29
5'1"	112 to 152	3 to 5	5'7"	148 to 188	3 to 5
	152 to 192	6 to 13		188 to 228	6 to 13
	192 to 232	14 to 21		228 to 268	14 to 21
	232 to 272	22 to 29		268 to 308	22 to 29
5'2"	118 to 158	3 to 5	5'8"	154 to 194	3 to 5
	158 to 198	6 to 13		194 to 234	6 to 13
	198 to 238	14 to 21		234 to 274	14 to 21
	238 to 278	22 to 29		274 to 314	22 to 29
5'3"	124 to 164	3 to 5	5'9"	160 to 200	3 to 5
	164 to 204	6 to 13		200 to 240	6 to 13
	204 to 244	14 to 21		240 to 280	14 to 21
	244 to 284	22 to 29		280 to 320	22 to 29
5'4"	130 to 170	3 to 5	5'10"	166 to 206	3 to 5
	170 to 210	6 to 13		206 to 246	6 to 13
	210 to 250	14 to 21		246 to 286	14 to 21
	250 to 290	22 to 29		286 to 326	22 to 29
5'5"	136 to 176	3 to 5	5'11"	172 to 212	3 to 5
	176 to 216	6 to 13		212 to 252	6 to 13
	216 to 256	14 to 21		252 to 292	14 to 21
	256 to 296	22 to 29		292 to 332	22 to 29

Height	Weight at start of 8 weeks	Expected fat loss in pounds/inches after 8 weeks plus slip-ups
6'0"	178 to 218	3 to 5
	218 to 258	6 to 13
	258 to 298	14 to 21
	298 to 338	22 to 29
6'1"	184 to 224	3 to 5
	224 to 264	6 to 13
	264 to 304	14 to 21
	304 to 344	22 to 29
6'2"	190 to 230	3 to 5
	230 to 270	6 to 13
	270 to 310	14 to 21
	310 to 350	22 to 29
6'3"	196 to 236	3 to 5
	236 to 276	6 to 13
	276 to 316	14 to 21
	316 to 356	22 to 29
6'4"	202 to 242	3 to 5
	242 to 282	6 to 13
	282 to 322	14 to 21
	322 to 363	22 to 29
6'5"	208 to 248	3 to 5
	248 to 288	6 to 13
	288 to 328	14 to 21
	328 to 368	22 to 29
6'6"	214 to 254	3 to 5
	254 to 294	6 to 13
	294 to 334	14 to 21
	334 to 374	22 to 29

Notes

Introduction

1. National Institute of Diabetes and Digestive and Kidney Diseases, "Overweight and Obesity Statistics," www.niddk.nih.gov/health-information/health-statistics/Pages/overweight-obesity-statistics.aspx.

2. Maggie Hennessy, "Americans' Eating Habits Worst Since 2008; 'Systemic Change' Needed, RD Says," Food Navigator-USA.com, December 6, 2013, www.foodnavigator-usa.com/Markets/Americans-eating-habits-worst-since-2008-systemic-change-needed-RD-says.

3. Harriet Brown, "The Weight of Evidence," Slate, March 24, 2015, www.slate.com/articles/health_and_science/medical_examiner/2015/03/diets_do_not_work_the_thin_evidence_that_losing_weight_makes_you_healthier.html.

Chapter 1. A Proven Program to Change Your Life

1. "Metabolic Syndrome: The Fat Disease," CBSNews, January 15, 2002, www.cbsnews.com/news/metabolic-syndrome-the-fat-disease.

2. "Metabolic Syndrome," MedicineNet.com, www.medicinenet.com/metabolic_syndrome/article.htm, June 2, 2015.

Chapter 3. Understanding Your Unique Metabolism

1. Teri L. Hernandez, John M. Kittelson, Christopher K. Law, Lawrence L. Ketch, Nicole R. Stob, Rachel C. Lindstrom, Ann Scherzinger, Elizabeth R. Stamm, and Robert H. Eckel, "Fat Redistribution Following Suction Lipectomy: Defense of Body Fat and Patterns of Restoration," Obesity 19, no. 7 (April 2011): 1388–1395.

Chapter 4. What Happened? Other Diets Used to Work for Me

1. Martin Reinhardt, Marie S. Thearly, Mostafa Ibrahim, Maximilian G. Hohenadel, Clifton Bogardus, Jonathan Krakoff, and Susanne B. Votruba, "A

Human Thrifty Phenotype Associated with Less Weight Loss During Caloric Restriction," *Diabetes* 64, no. 8 (August 2015): 2859–2867.

Chapter 14. Breast Cancer and Met B

1. M. J. Gunter, D. R. Hoover, H. Yu, S Wassertheil-Smoller, T. E. Rohan, J. E. Manson, J. Li et al., "Insulin, Insulin-Like Growth Factor-I, and Risk of Breast Cancer in Postmenopausal Women," *Journal of the National Cancer Institute* 101, no. 1 (January 2009): 48–60.

2. M. J. Gunter, X. Xie, X. Xue, G. C. Kabat, T. E. Rohan, S. Wassertheil-Smoller et al., "Breast Cancer Risk in Metabolically Healthy but Overweight Postmenopausal Women," *Cancer Research* 75, no. 2 (January 2015): 270–274.

3. Samy L. Habib and Maciej Rojna, "Diabetes and Risk of Cancer," *ISRN Oncology* 2013, no. 45 (2013): 1–16.

Chapter 16. High Cholesterol and Statins

1. Mayo Clinic, "Statins: Are These Cholesterol-Lowering Drugs Right for You?" www.mayoclinic.org/diseases-conditions/high-blood-cholesterol/in-depth/statins/art-20045772.

Glossary

ANXIETY, PANIC DISORDER: Many patients with Metabolism B report feelings of anxiety and nervousness that come and go. Some describe anxiety escalating to the point of panic attacks that can cause shortness of breath, pounding or rapid heartbeat, cold sweats, dizziness, fainting, and shakiness. Although panic attacks exist for many reasons, there is definitely a relationship between panic attacks and blood sugar fluctuations. Treatment for blood sugar panic attacks would require stabilizing the blood sugar.

ATTENTION DEFICIT DISORDER, OR ATTENTION-DEFICIT/HYPERACTIVITY DISORDER: ADD/ADHD is a neurobehavioral disorder. The Centers for Disease Control (CDC) estimates that approximately 11 percent of children ages four to seventeen (6.4 million) have been diagnosed with ADHD as of 2011.

- The percentage of children with an ADHD diagnosis continues to increase, from 7.8 percent in 2003 to 9.5 percent in 2007 and to 11.0 percent in 2011.
- Boys (13.2 percent) were more likely than girls (5.6 percent) to have ever been diagnosed with ADHD.
- The average age of children when receiving their ADHD diagnosis was seven, but children reported by their parents as having more severe ADHD were diagnosed earlier.

Although it typically presents itself during childhood, ADD/ADHD can last into adulthood. This disorder is usually treated by a combination of medication, behavior and lifestyle modification, and counseling. Interestingly, many of the symptoms of ADD/ADHD are also the symptoms of progressing Metabolism B. It seems prudent to check the fasting blood glucose and lipids of children diagnosed with ADD/ADHD to see whether changes in diet might help.

BLOOD GLUCOSE: Also known as blood sugar, blood glucose is the body's fuel. The amount of glucose in the blood varies throughout the day and is hormonally regulated by the pancreas with insulin and glucagon. Normal blood glucose is 65 to 140 mg/dL (3.6 to 7.8 mmol/L). Blood glucose can be stored as glycogen in the muscles and liver. Excesses of blood glucose (once the muscles and liver are refilled and circulating blood glucose is normalized) is stored as fat. Rises in blood glucose trigger the release of the fat-gain hormone, insulin. Low blood glucose triggers the release of glucagon.

BLOOD PRESSURE

hypertension (high blood pressure): Blood pressure consists of two readings: The upper reading, systolic, is the pressure created when your heart beats. It is considered high if it exceeds 140 mmHg. The lower reading, diastolic, is the measure of the pressure inside your blood vessels when the heart is at rest. It is considered elevated if it exceeds 90 mmHg. Hypertension is directly related to excess weight. For those with untreated Metabolism B, continual, gradual weight gain is a matter of fact. As weight increases, so too does blood pressure. The permanent weight loss effected by MM will quickly help decrease blood pressure.

The current blood pressure categories from the Mayo Clinic are:

normal blood pressure: Your blood pressure is normal if it's below 120/80 mmHg.

prehypertension: Prehypertension is a systolic pressure ranging from 120 to 139 mmHg or a diastolic pressure ranging from 80 to 89 mmHg. Prehypertension tends to get worse over time.

stage 1 hypertension: Stage 1 hypertension is a systolic pressure ranging from 140 to 159 mmHg or a diastolic pressure ranging from 90 to 99 mmHg.

stage 2 hypertension: More severe hypertension, stage 2 hypertension is a systolic pressure of 160 mmHg or higher or a diastolic pressure of 100 mmHg or higher.

CARBOHYDRATE: One of three major nutrients found in many foods like fruit, bread, legumes, milk, starchy veggies, potatoes, rice, and pasta as well as sweets, desserts, juice, soda, and chips. All carbohydrate converts into blood glucose and is the body's preferred fuel source.

CHRONIC FATIGUE: Also known as chronic fatigue syndrome, this type of exhaustion is an all-encompassing, draining fatigue often accompanied with aches and pains. The person with CFS wakes up tired and remains drained throughout much of the day, making everyday life activities a struggle. People use the terms "washed out" or "totally drained" to describe this exhaustion.

Metabolism B may be the cause of some CFS. If a person with CFS has Met B and follows the Metabolism Miracle, much of their fatigue, aches, and pains will be eliminated.

DEPRESSION (MILD): Depression is a medical condition involving an imbalance of brain chemistry. It is not diagnosed by a blood test but by the symptoms the patient relates to the physician or therapist.

If a person's glucose level has sharp peaks and valleys, it causes many of the same symptoms related to chemical depression. Because the symptoms of uncontrolled Met B and mild depression are so similar, depression related to blood glucose imbalance is often misdiagnosed as chemical depression and is unnecessarily treated with antidepressant medications; these are the patients who report little or no improvement in mild depression, even after their physician has changed the type or dose of antidepressant. Unfortunately it is not commonly accepted that blood glucose imbalance can mimic the symptoms of brain chemical imbalance. It is probably prudent to check a patient's blood glucose level as part of a medical evaluation for depression. If fasting blood glucose exceeds 85 mg/dL (4.7 mmol/L), the Metabolism Miracle lifestyle program should be recommended (perhaps initially MM in tandem with antidepressant medication).

DIABETES

prediabetes: Also known as borderline diabetes, prediabetes is a reversible condition. The diagnosis, made when fasting blood glucose is 100 to 125 mg/dL (5.6 to 6.9 mmol/L), is often considered a red flag that the patient is on the road to type 2 diabetes. With proper diet, exercise, and stress reduction, a diagnosis of type 2 diabetes may be prevented or forestalled. In an effort to be proactive, the Metabolism Miracle sets the bar for prediabetes at the lower range: 90 to 125 mg/dL (5 to 6.9 mmol/L).

type 2 diabetes: Type 2 diabetes is the most common form of diabetes and is caused by a genetic compilation and life stressors that cause either the pancreas to underproduce insulin and/or the insulin to progressively become resistant to fitting into cell receptors (insulin resistance). Insulin is necessary for the body to obtain glucose for energy; it is the "key" that opens the cells so they can accept glucose from the bloodstream. If the pancreas does not produce enough insulin or if the insulin can't open the cells appropriately, circulating glucose has nowhere to go and will build up in the bloodstream.

Type 2 diabetes is diagnosed with two fasting blood glucose tests over 125 mg/dL (6.9 mmol/L) or a high fasting blood glucose and hemoglobin A1C over

6.5. Recurrent elevations of blood glucose can, over time, damage blood vessels and nerves, leading to irreversible complications involving the eyes, nerves, kidneys, blood vessels, brain, and circulation.

type 1 diabetes: An autoimmune disease that results in the permanent destruction of the insulin-producing beta cells in the pancreas, type 1 diabetes's exact cause is unknown, but there appears to be a genetic link that may be precipitated by a virus, environmental toxin, illness, or stress. Previously known as juvenile diabetes, its onset is usually abrupt. It is often diagnosed in children and young adults, but it can occur at any age. It results in the absence of insulin, and people with type 1 diabetes currently require insulin administration for life.

gestational diabetes (GDM): GDM occurs in a pregnant woman who has never before had a diagnosis of diabetes but develops high blood glucose during the pregnancy. The normal placental hormones block the action of the mother's insulin. The pancreas fails to produce adequate insulin to bring the mother's blood glucose into normal range during the pregnancy. The treatment for GDM is diet modification, exercise as directed, and, in some cases, insulin injections. Most glucose levels normalize very soon after delivery. Babies born to mothers with untreated gestational diabetes often weigh close to nine pounds or more.

Gestational diabetes is routinely screened between weeks 24 and 28 of pregnancy with a fasting blood glucose and possibly an oral glucose tolerance test. Approximately 6 percent of pregnant women develop GDM. Women with a history of GDM have a greater chance of a recurrence during future pregnancies and of developing type 2 diabetes in the future.

FASTING BLOOD GLUCOSE: Fasting blood glucose is determined by a lab test drawn first thing in the morning after at least eight hours without food or calorie-containing beverages. This test can be used to determine blood glucose conditions including prediabetes or type 2 diabetes. The American Diabetes Association specifies normal fasting blood glucose level as 65 to 99 mg/dL (3.6 to 5.5 mmol/L), prediabetes as 100 to 125 mg/dL (5.6 to 6.9 mmol/L) (inclusive), and diabetes as 125 mg/dl (7 mmol/L) or higher. The diagnosis of diabetes should be confirmed with a second fasting blood glucose result greater than or equal to 126 mg/dL.

FAT CELLS: The number of fat cells you will carry throughout life is determined in utero and can increase at the beginning of puberty. When an adult gains weight, it is the size and not the number of fat cells that increases.

FIBROMYALGIA: This constellation of symptoms includes fatigue, muscle pain, and stiffness. It also can include constipation, headaches, decreased short-term memory and the ability to focus thoughts, menstrual cramping, numbness, tingling, dizziness, and skin sensitivity. Many of these symptoms overlap with the symptoms of chronic fatigue syndrome, insulin resistance, metabolic syndrome, prediabetes, hypoglycemia, and type 2 diabetes. These symptoms markedly improve for many people with Metabolism B who live the MM lifestyle.

GASTRIC REFLUX DISEASE (GERD): GERD can occur in people who have a hiatal hernia. Similar to the way increased midline fat can affect sleep apnea, the extra fat stores around the middle can press on the stomach and cause stomach acid to backflow into the esophagus. Weight loss around the middle drastically improves GERD's symptoms.

GLUCAGON: A pancreatic hormone that signals the liver to release glycogen stores and effectively helps increase blood glucose when it falls below normal. It begins the liver's self-feeding mechanism when we exceed four to five hours without carbohydrate intake.

GLYCEMIC INDEX: Also referred to as GI, this is an index that ranks carbohydrates based on the speed at which they convert to blood glucose. The glycemic index has a scale of 0 to 100, with the higher values given to foods that cause the most rapid rise in blood sugar. Pure glucose is the reference point, and it is given a GI of 100. For simple comparison, the foods are ranked according to their same size in weight, 50 grams. It is important to note, however, that the GI is not based on a typical portion size of food (see GLYCEMIC LOAD).

GLYCEMIC LOAD: GL ranks the glycemic index of foods according to the "typical" portion size of that particular food.

GLYCOGEN: Glycogen is stored glucose in muscle cells and liver. Glycogen is released from the muscles when a person exercises and is released from the liver if a person skips or delays a meal or during the sleep hours. When glycogen is released, it causes blood glucose to rise into or over the normal range.

HUNGER: Hunger is a natural physical phenomenon. It is an unpleasant feeling experienced when one's blood sugar level begins to drop four to five hours after a meal or when the glycogen stores in the muscle and liver drop below a certain threshold. The feeling associated with hunger gives us the desire to eat.

HYPOGLYCEMIA: There are two main types of hypoglycemia (blood glucose that is below normal). One is caused by excess insulin production and release for those with uncontrolled Met B. The other is drug induced from excess glucose-lowering medication for diabetes. This temporary state of low blood sugar comes with a complement of symptoms including shaking, light-headedness, confusion, irritability, hunger, carb cravings, cold sweats, and headache. Eating quick-acting carbohydrate foods and beverages immediately relieves the symptoms by causing a quick surge in blood glucose.

Hypoglycemia is generally classified when blood sugar dips below 70 mg/dL (3.9 mmol/L). Related to uncontrolled Met B, these symptoms can occur one and a half to two hours after a meal, when the overactive pancreas releases excess insulin. A person with normal metabolism should not experience hypoglycemia. (For treatment of hypoglycemia, see Chapter 12, page 232.)

HYPOTHYROIDISM: Thyroid hormones regulate the speed of metabolism. When the thyroid gland can't produce enough hormones, the metabolic rate slows. Symptoms include fatigue, weakness, weight gain, malaise, and difficulty losing weight. Dry skin, constipation, hair loss, muscle cramps, cold intolerance, depression, irritability, memory loss, abnormal menstrual cycles, and depressed libido can also be related to hypothyroidism. Many of the symptoms for insulin resistance, uncontrolled Met B, prediabetes, and type 2 diabetes are the same. Simple blood tests are used to determine whether thyroid hormone and glucose levels are normal. Only through blood tests can one determine hypothyroidism or blood glucose abnormalities.

INJECTABLE INSULIN: Used as a medical treatment for diabetes, injectable insulin is manufactured in the laboratory using recombinant DNA.

INSULIN: The hormone insulin, produced by the pancreas, helps *lower* blood glucose. Insulin acts like a key and opens the doorways into your fat and muscle cells, allowing excess glucose in your blood to move into the opened fat and muscle cells. This movement brings blood glucose back into the normal range and enables the glucose to be used for energy (muscle cells) or stored as fat (fat cells). Insulin is a storage hormone.

INSULIN RESISTANCE (IR): Insulin resistance occurs when the normal amount of insulin secreted by the pancreas is not able to work effectively. When insulin does not "fit" the cell's receptors appropriately, it cannot do its job to "open" the cell to receive excess glucose from the blood. Eventually the pancreas cannot keep up with the body's need for insulin, and excess glucose builds up in the bloodstream. Ironically, many people with insulin resistance have high levels of blood glucose and high levels of insulin circulating in their blood at the same time.

LIVER: The liver contains a stockpile of blood glucose in the form of glycogen. When you skip or delay a meal, as well as every night while you are asleep, it is the liver's release of glycogen that keeps your body working. Through the liver's intervention the human body has the ability to "self-feed."

METABOLIC SYNDROME: This group of conditions increases your risk for diabetes, heart disease, and stroke. Symptoms include gaining fat around the middle, increased blood pressure, elevated insulin levels, excess body fat around the waist, elevated LDL cholesterol, elevated triglycerides, decreased HDL cholesterol, prediabetes, and type 2 diabetes. A major root cause of metabolic syndrome is insulin imbalance and insulin resistance.

MIDLINE FAT DEPOSITS: One of the hallmarks of insulin imbalance in Met B is a growing roll of fat around the middle. Some people also note increased "back fat." This hallmark fat deposit around the middle even occurs in otherwise thin patients.

NET CARBOHYDRATE: The amount of carbohydrate that will eventually convert to blood glucose. Net carbohydrate is *included* in the total carbohydrate grams on a food label. Use the following formula to determine net carbs:

Total carbohydrate grams – dietary fiber grams = net carbohydrate grams

Never subtract sugar alcohol from total carbohydrate to find a net carb, as a portion of sugar alcohol grams will convert to blood glucose. (The only sugar alcohol that should be subtracted from the total carb grams is erythritol.)

NORMAL BLOOD GLUCOSE RANGE: A person with normal carbohydrate metabolism will have blood glucose between 65 and 140 mg/dL (3.6 and 7.8 mmol/L), regardless of what he or she chooses to eat or not eat. In terms of normal blood glucose metabolism, a person can choose to fast for two days or eat a half-pound of pasta with a loaf of garlic bread, and in either case his or her blood glucose will remain in the 65 to 140 mg/dL range. Blood glucose is hormonally regulated by the pancreas with the help of the hormones insulin and glucagon.

OSTEOARTHRITIS (OA): An inflammatory condition with decreased lubricating fluid in the joints that causes abnormal wearing of the protective cartilage that covers the joints. As the protection of the joints decreases, simple activities such as walking and standing become painful. Activity usually decreases, and inactivity can compromise the functioning of muscles and ligaments. Increased body weight caused by uncontrolled Met B causes osteoarthritis to be more painful and to progress faster.

OSTEOPENIA: Osteopenia occurs when bone density dips below normal. Regular exercise along with calcium and vitamin D supplementation help to alleviate the problem. Physical activity can also help with bone density. Being overweight and inactive with a deficiency of vitamin D (as in uncontrolled Met B) can lead to osteoporosis.

OSTEOPOROSIS: In this disease bone mineral density is so compromised that an increased risk of bone fracture results. Hypothyroidism and type 2 diabetes contribute to the condition. Regular exercise, along with calcium and vitamin D supplementation, helps to prevent the condition.

PANCREAS: The dual-function gland/organ responsible for producing hormones that regulate blood sugar (insulin and glucagon) and digestive enzymes. Insulin and glucagon keep blood glucose in the normal range of 65 to 140 mg/dL (3.6 to 7.8 mmol/L) throughout the day and night.

POLYCYSTIC OVARIAN SYNDROME (PCOS): This endocrine disorder affects more than 10 percent of all women. Possibly caused by insulin resistance and the genes related to type 2 diabetes, its symptoms include:

- hirsutism (excessive hair growth on the face, chest, abdomen, etc.)
- hair loss in a classic "male baldness" pattern
- acne
- polycystic ovaries
- obesity with weight gain around the middle
- infertility or reduced fertility

In addition, women with PCOS appear to be at increased risk of developing the following health problems during their lives:

- insulin resistance
- diabetes
- lipid abnormalities
- obstructive sleep apnea
- cardiovascular disease
- endometrial carcinoma (cancer)

Not all women with PCOS have all the symptoms. Almost all have insulin resistance (uncontrolled Met B). Women with the disorder do not ovulate in a predictable manner and also produce excessive quantities of androgens, particularly testosterone. They have an increased risk of diabetes, LDL, HDL, and triglyceride abnormalities, sleep apnea, cardiovascular disease, endometriosis, and endometrial cancer.

SLEEP APNEA: In this sleep disorder long pauses in breathing during sleep cause people to miss a number of breaths throughout the night. Weight loss helps with the loud snoring and restless sleep, and the daytime fatigue that accompanies sleep apnea. Untreated Metabolism B accumulates fat around the middle, which puts pressure on the diaphragm during sleep. The Metabolism Miracle's fat-burning steps decrease midline fat and help decrease pressure on the diaphragm, thereby helping to alleviate sleep apnea.

SLEEP DISTURBANCE: Two different sleep disturbances occur with uncontrolled Metabolism B. One is the brain's inability to relax and allow the person to fall asleep, even when the body is legitimately tired. The other disturbance occurs when a person falls asleep easily, awakens in the middle of the night, and cannot return to sleep. Both sleep disturbances seem to be caused by peaks and valleys of blood glucose during the night.

Acknowledgments

PHIL KRESEFSKI SR., my lifetime sweetheart. We've been together for over forty years and married for over thirty-three. Walking life's path together has been a journey, including high mountains and deep valleys. We're still holding hands.

Thank you, Phil, for encouraging me to write *The Metabolism Miracle, Second Edition*. You kept me going by reminding me of basic needs by saying things like, "You have to eat—you have Met B," bringing me water and decaf drinks until I exceeded sixty-four ounces, putting out vitamins and supplements, making my green tea, and ensuring I got some early morning sunshine and daily exercise. You are my best friend, a great husband, and a wonderful father and grandfather to our children and grandchildren. Now we can have some fun!

JOHN RADZIEWICZ, publisher at DaCapo Press of Perseus Books. Thanks for answering my questions over the years. I "used to be" a feisty, strong-willed person, but you always made time for me to discuss issues and concerns. I'm still a feisty and strong-willed person, but now I'm one who calls you less often. I appreciate all you've done to make The Metabolism Miracle series a reality. You've been wonderful to me and I appreciate it.

DAN AMBROSIO, senior editor at Perseus Books. This has been one heck of a ride. But in the end the second edition is here, and you made it possible to update the program and give MM followers an up-to-date book with all the program tweaks and newest information.

CHRISTINE MARRA, the excellent detail-oriented editor who really cleaned and polished the book with professionalism. Yes, editing is a "Marrathon"—and Christine is a great talent.

ANDREA SOMBERG, my first ever literary agent at the Harvey Klinger Agency in New York City. Andrea saw promise in the original MM manuscript and connected me with my long-term publisher, Perseus Books.

We've come full circle, Andrea, and it's been a colorful and fascinating journey. Thank you.

DIANA AND JAY DONNELLY: Diana, thanks for being my favorite daughter and best friend. Thank you both for my dear grandchildren, Jason (JJ) and Joseph (Joey). "I'm reasonably certain they will be president and vice president one day," says their very biased grandma . . . XOXO.

PHILLIP KRESEFSKI JR. AND HIS FIANCÉE, JEN LATONDRESS. Phillip, you are my big softy. We've spent lots of fun times together as I wrote this book, especially when you temporarily took up residence in Florida. You're now many miles to the north and have joined Jen in starting your new life together. Thanks for reminding me what young love looks like. And Jen, you are a welcome addition to the annual family portrait at the beach!

RAYMOND KRESEFSKI SR., my father-in-law and all-around wonderful person. My "dad" was selfless, caring, and unconditionally loving. I miss you very much.

DEE GRAHL, administrator of Miracle-Ville.com and my dear friend. Thanks so much for walking with me along the MV journey and for your support, sense of humor, laughs, and long-distance problem solving. I appreciate you more than you know.

MEMBERS OF MIRACLE-VILLE.COM: a special thanks to all members of Miracle-Ville. I was away for a while as I focused attention on the new book. Thanks for working with Dee to help others on the site by sharing your recipes, advice, support, encouragement, and knowledge. I always feel at "home" in the 'Ville!

DAVID HANNA, thanks for being there during some major moments in my life. I enjoyed our chats when I wrote the first book and our fun times since. Wishing you a great life with many EDLPs.

Index

Hearty Sausage and Bean Soup, 289

caffeine, as diuretic, 174

carb charts, 148–150

carb-counting myth, 44–45, 48

Carb Dams, 116–126, 136–137, 139–140

carb range, identifying, 145–147

carb servings, 154, 162–164

carbohydrates
  bogus 5-gram Counter Carbs, 67–70
  "carb is a carb" myth, 44–45
  Counter Carbs, 62–64
  definition, 348
  net carb formula, 57, 64–67, 106, 117–119, 162–163
  net carb grams, 106, 164 (chart), 353
  overreaction to, xviii, 24–25, 113, 115, 119, 126, 147, 168
  reintroducing, 43–45, 113–116
  stacking, 62, 100, 103, 106, 116
  timed pattern of, 15

cardiovascular disease, 15

carrots
  Carrot Cake with Cream Cheese Frosting, 333–334
  Ham and Pineapple Chopped Salad with Side Wrap, 281
  Hearty Sausage and Bean Soup, 289
  Pasta Primavera Salad, 293
  Springtime Stir Fry, 300–301
  Veggie Couscous Soup, 287

cauliflower
  Buffalo "Wings," Cauliflower Style, 275
  Cauliflower Rice, 321
  "Faux" Mashed Potatoes, 318
  Miracle "Faux-Tato" Salad, 295
  Miracle "Potatoless" Soup, 286–287
  Pasta Primavera Salad, 293
  Potato-ish Salad, 291

Tropical Salsa Scallops, 302

Veggie Couscous Soup, 287

celebrity spokespeople, xvii

cheese
  Broccoli-Cheese Casserole, 317–318
  Cheddar Cheese Biscuits, 325–326
  Cheddar Flax Crackers, 326
  Cheesy Chips, 277
  Classic Pesto, 279
  Cold Salmon, Quinoa, and Asparagus Salad, 306–307
  Crispy Tortilla Chips, 276
  Crustless Ham, Cheddar, and Veggie Quiche, 264–265
  Easy "Bacon" Pizza, 267
  Easy Pizza, 266–267
  Egg Taco, 263
  Feta-Stuffed Mushrooms, 274–275
  Flavorful Turkey Burgers, 300
  Greek-Inspired Wraps, 280–281
  Miracle Grilled Cheese, 281–282
  Miracle "Potatoless" Soup, 286–287
  Miracle Zero-Carb Pasta, Turkey, and Veggie Bake, 298–299
  Neutral Pizza with Cream Cheese Crust, 309–310
  Philly Cheese Steak, 305
  Roasted Broccoli and Cheddar Soup, 285
  Sun-Dried Tomato Dip, 278
  Veggie Mini-Pizza, 274

chicken
  Chicken Paprikash, 302–303
  Chicken Salad with Curry, 296
  Chicken Scampi Miracle Pasta, 304
  Chunky Chicken Salad, 292
  Lemony Dill Chicken, 297–298
  Philly Cheese Steak, 305
  Springtime Stir Fry, 300–301

chickpeas
  Crockpot Chili, 311–312
  Open-Faced Hummus and Avocado, 282–283
  Three-Bean Salad, 294

children, 169–170

eating out, 216–221
eggplants
    All-Veggie Lasagna, 313–314
    Eggplant Rollatini, 312–313
eggs
    Chocolate-Dipped Chocolate
        Meringue Cookies, 339
    Chocolate Meringues, 338
    Crustless Ham, Cheddar, and
        Veggie Quiche, 264–265
    Easy Egg Cups, 261
    Egg Taco, 263
    Healthy "McMiracle" Muffin, 262
    Holiday Egg Nog, 323
    Light Chef's Salad, 290
    Miracle Quiche, 263–264
    Silver Dollar Pancakes, 269
    Spicy Salad, 294–295
    Sun-Dried Tomato and Spinach
        Omelet, 265
    Sunshine Breakfast Sandwich,
        262
    Tender Spinach Salad, 290–291
    Turkey Frittata, 314–315
entrées
    All-Veggie Lasagna, 313–314
    Breaded Baked Flounder, 307–308
    Chicken Paprikash, 302–303
    Chicken Scampi Miracle Pasta,
        304
    Cold Salmon, Quinoa, and
        Asparagus Salad, 306–307
    Crockpot Chili, 311–312
    Eggplant Rollatini, 312–313
    Flavorful Turkey Burgers, 300
    Lemony Dill Chicken, 297–298
    Miracle Zero-Carb Pasta, Turkey,
        and Veggie Bake, 298–299
    Neutral Pizza with Cream Cheese
        Crust, 309–310
    Open-Faced Portabello Cap
        Sandwich, 315
    Philly Cheese Steak, 305
    Seafood Delight, 306
    Shish Kebab, 308–309

    Spaghetti Squash "Spaghetti,"
        303–304
    Spicy Shrimp and Zucchini, 301
    Springtime Stir Fry, 300–301
    Stuffed Peppers, 316
    Swedish Meatballs, 310–311
    Tropical Salsa Scallops, 302
    Turkey Frittata, 314–315
    Whole-Wheat Pasta with Chicken
        Sausage Ragu, 299–300
erythritol, 69–70, 72
EU labels, 71
exercise
    activity levels, 147
    after a meal, 196–197
    amount per day, 57, 183, 185–186
    armchair, 188
    Fueling Forward, 121, 190–193
    importance of, 56, 105
    Metabolism B (Met B) and, 33
    monthly log (form), 194
    pre-exercise snack, 190, 195–196
    purpose of, 183
    skipping, 193, 195
    suggestions for moving, 189
    timing, 190, 193
    types, 187–188
    workout efficiency, 188, 190

fast food, 221
fasting insulin level test, 17–18
fat-burning, 57, 76
fat cells, 38–39, 112, 350
fat-free foods, 76, 83, 84
fat tissue compared to muscle tissue,
    184
fatigue, chronic, 13
fiber, 65, 139
fibromyalgia, 351
fish
    Breaded Baked Flounder, 307–308
    Cold Salmon, Quinoa, and
        Asparagus Salad, 306–307
    Nicoise "Sandwiches," 282
    Seafood Delight, 306

About the Author

Diane Kress, RD CDE, is a registered dietitian, certified diabetes educator, and person with type 2 diabetes. With over thirty-five years' experience in the field of medical nutrition therapy, she has focused her practice on diet and lifestyle therapy for those who struggle with excess weight, obesity, metabolic syndrome, prediabetes, type 2 diabetes, and pre- and post-weight-loss surgery.

After years of focusing on medical nutrition and directing the diet and diabetes centers in hospitals and medical centers, she researched and developed the proprietary program presented in this book. The Metabolism Miracle program is the result of years of research, development, fine tuning, and data collection at her private practice in Morristown, New Jersey, the Nutrition Center of Morristown.

Kress's program, the Metabolism Miracle, has already helped thousands of her private practice patients, clients, and readership from around the world who have lost weight and kept it off and now experience high energy, restful sleep, and improved focus and concentration while attaining and retaining weight loss, fat loss, and improved levels of blood glucose, HbA1C, cholesterol, triglycerides, blood pressure, vitamin D, and insulin.

She feels blessed to have been able to bring the Metabolism Miracle to the world.

Besides *The Metabolism Miracle,* she has written :

The Metabolism Miracle Cookbook

The Metabolism Miracle Deluxe Edition

The Diabetes Miracle

And now *The Metabolism Miracle, Second Edition*

Kress is an advocate for those who struggle with weight and weight-related medical conditions and experience progressively declining health and wellness.

She lives in Southwest Florida with her husband and near her children and grandchildren.

Blog: www.dianekress.wordpress.com
Metabolism Miracle's subscription support site:
   www.Miracle-Ville.com
Websites: www.themetabolismmiracle.com
            www.thediabetesmiracle.com
Social Media: Follow Diane Kress on Facebook, Twitter, LinkedIn,
   Pinterest, and Google Plus

Laughter is timeless, imagination has no age,
and dreams are forever.
— TINKERBELL